THE ROLE OF THE INTERNET OF THINGS (IoT) IN BIOMEDICAL ENGINEERING

Present Scenario and Challenges

Biomedical Engineering: Techniques and Applications Book Series

THE ROLE OF THE INTERNET OF THINGS (IoT) IN BIOMEDICAL ENGINEERING

Present Scenario and Challenges

Edited by

Sushree Bibhuprada B. Priyadarshini, PhD
Devendra Kumar Sharma, PhD
Rohit Sharma, PhD
Korhan Cengiz, PhD

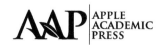

First edition published 2022

Apple Academic Press Inc.
1265 Goldenrod Circle, NE,
Palm Bay, FL 32905 USA

4164 Lakeshore Road, Burlington,
ON, L7L 1A4 Canada

CRC Press
6000 Broken Sound Parkway NW,
Suite 300, Boca Raton, FL 33487-2742 USA

2 Park Square, Milton Park,
Abingdon, Oxon, OX14 4RN UK

© 2022 by Apple Academic Press, Inc.

Apple Academic Press exclusively co-publishes with CRC Press, an imprint of Taylor & Francis Group, LLC

Reasonable efforts have been made to publish reliable data and information, but the authors, editors, and publisher cannot assume responsibility for the validity of all materials or the consequences of their use. The authors, editors, and publishers have attempted to trace the copyright holders of all material reproduced in this publication and apologize to copyright holders if permission to publish in this form has not been obtained. If any copyright material has not been acknowledged, please write and let us know so we may rectify in any future reprint.

Except as permitted under U.S. Copyright Law, no part of this book may be reprinted, reproduced, transmitted, or utilized in any form by any electronic, mechanical, or other means, now known or hereafter invented, including photocopying, microfilming, and recording, or in any information storage or retrieval system, without written permission from the publishers.

For permission to photocopy or use material electronically from this work, access www.copyright.com or contact the Copyright Clearance Center, Inc. (CCC), 222 Rosewood Drive, Danvers, MA 01923, 978-750-8400. For works that are not available on CCC please contact mpkbookspermissions@tandf.co.uk

Trademark notice: Product or corporate names may be trademarks or registered trademarks and are used only for identification and explanation without intent to infringe.

Library and Archives Canada Cataloguing in Publication

Title: The role of the Internet of Things (IoT) in biomedical engineering : present scenario and challenges / edited by Sushree Bibhuprada, B. Priyadarshini, PhD, Devendra Kumar Sharma, PhD, Rohit Sharma, PhD, Korhan Cengiz, PhD.
Names: Priyadarshini, Sushree Bibhuprada B., editor. | Sharma, Devendra Kumar, editor. | Sharma, Rohit (Assistant professor of electronics), editor. | Cengiz, Korhan, editor.
Series: Biomedical engineering (Apple Academic Press)
Description: First edition. | Series statement: Biomedical engineering: techniques and applications book series | Includes bibliographical references and index.
Identifiers: Canadiana (print) 20210317396 | Canadiana (ebook) 20210317426 | ISBN 9781774630129 (hardcover) | ISBN 9781774638736 (softcover) | ISBN 9781003180470 (ebook)
Subjects: LCSH: Biomedical engineering. | LCSH: Internet of things.
Classification: LCC R856 .R65 2022 | DDC 610.28—dc23

Library of Congress Cataloging-in-Publication Data

Names: Priyadarshini, Sushree Bibhuprada B., editor. | Sharma, Devendra Kumar, editor. | Sharma, Rohit (Assistant professor of electronics). editor. | Cengiz, Korhan, editor.
Title: The role of Internet of Things (IoT) in biomedical engineering : present scenario and challenges / edited by Sushree Bibhuprada B. Priyadarshini, Devendra Kumar Sharma, Rohit Sharma, Korhan Cengiz.
Other titles: Role of the Internet of Things (IoT) in biomedical engineering | Biomedical engineering (Apple Academic Press)
Description: 1st edition. | Palm Bay, FL : Apple Academic Press, Inc., 2022. | Series: Biomedical engineering: techniques and applications book series | Includes bibliographical references and index. | Summary: "This volume introduces the key evolving applications of IoT in the medical field for patient care delivery through the usage of smart devices. It shows how IoT opens the door to a wealth of relevant healthcare information through real-time data analysis as well as testing, providing reliable and pragmatic data that yields enhanced solutions and discovery of previously undiscovered issues. The Role of the Internet of Things (IoT) in Biomedical Engineering: Present Scenario and Challenges discusses IoT devices that are deployed for enabling patient health tracking, various emergency issues, smart administration of patients, etc. It looks at the problems of cardiac analysis in e-healthcare, explores the employment of smart devices aimed for different patient issues, and examines the usage of Arduino kits where the data can be transferred to cloud for internet-based uses. The volume also considers the roles of IoT in electroencephalography (EEG) and magnetic resonance imaging (MRI), which play significant roles in biomedical applications. This book also incorporates the use of IoT applications for smart wheelchairs, telemedicine, GPS positioning of heart patients, smart administration with drug tracking, and more. Key features: Explores the use of IoT in the field of biomedical engineering Discusses current issues associated with biomedical engineering while including the fundamentals such as collaboration on usage of sensors, bio-interfaces, e-medicine, remote healthcare, etc. Throws light on IoT for healthcare monitoring as well as for remote healthcare, data communication, monitoring, and diagnosis. The book will help readers to keep abreast of the current novel technologies for conducting research while employing various diagnostic tools and to explore frontiers of what is realizable in practice"-- Provided by publisher.
Identifiers: LCCN 2021045070 (print) | LCCN 2021045071 (ebook) | ISBN 9781774630129 (hardback) | ISBN 9781774638736 (paperback) | ISBN 9781003180470 (ebook)
Subjects: MESH: Biomedical Engineering | Internet of Things | Medical Informatics Applications | Telemedicine
Classification: LCC R856.15 (print) | LCC R856.15 (ebook) | NLM QT 36 | DDC 610.28--dc23
LC record available at https://lccn.loc.gov/2021045070
LC ebook record available at https://lccn.loc.gov/2021045071

ISBN: 978-1-77463-012-9 (hbk)
ISBN: 978-1-77463-873-6 (pbk)
ISBN: 978-1-00318-047-0 (ebk)

ABOUT THE BOOK SERIES BIOMEDICAL ENGINEERING: TECHNIQUES AND APPLICATIONS

This new book series covers important research issues and concepts of the biomedical engineering progress in alignment with the latest technologies and applications. The books in the series include chapters on the recent research developments in the field of biomedical engineering. The series explores various real-time/offline medical applications that directly or indirectly rely on medical and information technology. Books in the series include case studies in the fields of medical science, i.e., biomedical engineering, medical information security, interdisciplinary tools along with modern tools, and technologies used.

Coverage & Approach

- In-depth information about biomedical engineering along with applications.
- Technical approaches in solving real-time health problems
- Practical solutions through case studies in biomedical data
- Health and medical data collection, monitoring, and security

The editors welcome book chapters and book proposals on all topics in the biomedical engineering and associated domains, including Big Data, IoT, ML, and emerging trends and research opportunities.

BOOK SERIES EDITORS:

Raghvendra Kumar, PhD
Associate Professor, Computer Science & Engineering Department,
GIET University, India
Email: raghvendraagrawal7@gmail.com

Vijender Kumar Solanki, PhD
Associate Professor, Department of CSE,
CMR Institute of Technology (Autonomous), Hyderabad, India
Email: spesinfo@yahoo.com

Noor Zaman, PhD
School of Computing and Information Technology,
Taylor's University, Selangor, Malaysia
Email: noorzaman650@hotmail.com

Brojo Kishore Mishra, PhD
Professor, Department of CSE, School of Engineering,
GIET University, Gunupur, Odisha, India
Email: bkmishra@giet.edu

FORTHCOMING BOOKS IN THE SERIES

Handbook of Artificial Intelligence in Biomedical Engineering
Editors: Saravanan Krishnan, Ramesh Kesavan, and B. Surendiran

Handbook of Deep Learning in Biomedical Engineering and Health Informatics
Editors: E. Golden Julie, S. M. Jai Sakthi, and Harold Y. Robinson

Biomedical Devices for Different Health Applications
Editors: Garima Srivastava and Manju Khari

Handbook of Research on Emerging Paradigms for Biomedical and Rehabilitation Engineering
Editors: Manuel Cardona and Cecilia García Cena

High-Performance Medical Image Processing
Editors: Sanjay Saxena and Sudip Paul

ABOUT THE EDITORS

Sushree Bibhuprada B. Priyadarshini, PhD (Computer Science and Engineering), is Assistant Professor in the Department of Computer Science and Information Technology at the Institute of Technical Education and Research (ITER), Siksha 'O' Anusandhan, Deemed to be University, India. She is a recipient of an Orissa State Talent Scholarship and NRTS Scholarship. She has been awarded a Best Poster Presentation at the workshop on Monitoring of Research of PhD Scholars (MRS–2017) at VSSUT, Burla (An Event of Diamond Jubilee Celebration 1956–2016). She has received a Best Student Paper Award at the 15th International Conference on Information Technology, IEEE, organized by IIIT, Bhubaneswar, in 2016. She has been awarded a Best Poster Presentation Award at a workshop on Women in Smart Computing, organized at KIIT, Bhubaneswar, in 2017. She has been invited and selected as the Keynote Speaker at the International Conference of Innovative Applied Energy, St. Cross College, Oxford University, UK. In addition, she is a member of several organizations, including IAENG, SDIWC, and CSTA. She is also working as reviewer for *the International Journal of Engineering Research & Technology* and *IEEE Consumer Electronics Journal.* She has published over 25 papers in various international journals and conferences, including IET, IEEE, Elsevier, Springer, IGI Global, etc.

Devendra Kumar Sharma, PhD, received his B.E. degree in Electronics Engineering from Motilal Nehru National Institute of Technology, Allahabad in 1989, M.E degree from Indian Institute of Technology Roorkee, Roorkee in 1992 and PhD degree from National Institute of Technology, Kurukshetra, India in 2016. He served PSU in different positions for more than 8 years in QA & Testing / R & D departments. Dr. Sharma joined the department of Electronics and Communication Engineering, Meerut Institute of Engineering and Technology, Meerut, Uttar Pradesh, India in October 2000 as Senior Lecturer and worked there till April 2018 at different capacities of Assistant Professor, Associate Professor, Professor and Dean Academics. He is currently working a Professor and Dean of SRM Institute of Science and Technology, Delhi-NCR Campus,

Ghaziabad, India. Dr. Sharma has authored many papers in several international journals and conferences of repute. His research interests include VLSI interconnects, Electronic Circuits, Digital Design, Testing and Signal Processing. He is a reviewer of many international journals belonging to various publication houses such as IEEE, Elsevier, Emerald, World Scientific, and Springer. Dr. Sharma has participated in many International and National conferences as Session Chair, and member of Steering, Advisory and Technical Program Committees. He has been the Editor for several books / conference proceedings and has been the Organizing Chair for several international conferences. He is life member of ISTE, Fellow of IETE and Senior Member of IEEE.

Rohit Sharma, PhD, is Assistant Professor in the Department of Electronics and Communication Engineering, SRM Institute of Science and Technology, Delhi NCR Campus Ghaziabad, India. He earned his PhD at Teerthanker Mahaveer University, Moradabad, India. He is an active member of ISTE, IEEE, ICS, IAENG, and IACSIT. He is an editorial board member and reviewer of several international journals and conferences. He has published about 36 research papers in international and national journals and about nine research papers in international and national conferences. Dr. Sharma has participated in many international and national conferences as session chair and as a member of the steering, advisory, and international program committees.

Korhan Cengiz, PhD, is Assistant Professor in the Department of Telecommunication at Trakya University, Trakya, Edirne, Turkey. Dr. Cengiz has published more than 30 articles related to wireless sensor networks and wireless communications. He services as a TPC member more than 20 conferences. He is editor-in-chief of two journals and editor of several journals. His honors include a Tubitak Priority Areas PhD scholarship and two best paper awards at conferences: ICAT 2016 and ICAT 2018. He received his BS degree in Electronics and Communication Engineering from Kocaeli University, Turkey. He received his PhD degree in Electronics Engineering from Kadir Has University, Turkey.

CONTENTS

Contributors xi
Abbreviations xiii
Preface xvii

1. **Use of IoT in Biomedical Signal Analysis for Healthcare Systems** 1
   Mihir Narayan Mohanty, Saumendra Kumar Mohapatra, and
   Mohan Debarchan Mohanty

2. **Application of the Internet of Things (IoT) for Biomedical
   Peregrination and Smart Healthcare** 31
   Aradhana Behura and Sushree Bibhuprada B. Priyadarshini

3. **Analysis of Efficiencies between EEG and MRI: A Survey** 69
   Namrata P. Mohanty, Sweta Shree Dash, and Tripti Swarnkar

4. **A State-of-the-Art Survey on Decision Trees in the Context of
   Big Data Analysis and IoT** 99
   Monalisa Jena and Satchidananda Dehuri

5. **The Emerging Role of The Internet of Things (IoT) in the
   Biomedical Industry** 129
   Amrit Sahani and Sushree Bibhuprada B. Priyadarshini

6. **A Comprehensive Survey on the Internet of Things (IoT)
   in Healthcare** 157
   Deepak Garg, Devendra Kumar Sharma, Prashant Mani, and Brajesh Kumar Kaushik

7. **Odontogenic Tumors: Prevalence and Demographic
   Distribution through IoT** 185
   Priyanka Debta, Sibani Sarangi, Debabrata Singh, Anurag Dani,
   Somalee Mahapatra, and Mitrabinda Khuntia

8. **Relevant Current Applications of the Internet of Things (IoT)
   in Biomedical Engineering** 207
   Anish Kumar

Index 249

CONTRIBUTORS

Aradhana Behura
Veer Surendra Sai University of Technology, Burla, India. E-mail: aradhanabehura@gmail.com

Anurag Dani
Department of Prosthodontia, C.D.C.R.I. Rajnandgaon, Chhattisgarh, India

Sweta Shree Dash
Department of Computer Science & Engg, Siksha 'O' Anusandhan (Deemed to be University), Bhubaneswar, India. E-mail: sweta.soa@gmail.com

Priyanka Debta
I.D.S, Siksha "O" Anusandhan, (Deemed to be University), Bhubaneswar, India

Satchidananda Dehuri
P.G. Department of I &CT, Fakir Mohan University, Balasore, India. E-mail: satchi.lapa@gmail.com

Deepak Garg
Department of Electronics and Communication Engineering, IIMT Engineering College, Meerut, India.
E-mail: deepakgarg1985@gmail.com

Monalisa Jena
P.G. Department of I & CT, Fakir Mohan University, Balasore, India. E-mail: bmonalisa.26@gmail.com

Brajesh Kumar Kaushik
Department of Electronics and Communication Engineering, IIT-Roorkee, Roorkee, India.
E-mail: bkkaushik23@gmail.com

Mitrabinda Khuntia
ITER, Department of CSE, Siksha "O" Anusandhan, (Deemed to be University),
Hitech Dental College & Hospitals, Bhubaneswar, India

Anish Kumar
Computer Science and Information Technology, Institute of Technical Education and Research (ITER), Siksha 'O' Anusandhan (Deemed to be University), Bhubaneswar, India.
E-mail: anishkumar2159@gmail.com

Somalee Mahapatra
Department of Pathology and Microbiology, Hitech Dental College& Hospitals, Bhubaneswar, India.
E-mail: debabratasingh@soa.ac.in

Prashant Mani
Department of Electronics and Communication Engineering, IIMT Engineering College, SRM-IST, Ghaziabad, India. E-mail: prashantmani29@gmail.com

Mihir Narayan Mohanty
ITER, Siksha 'O' Anusandhan (Deemed to be University), Bhubaneswar, India.
E-mail: mihir.n.mohanty@gmail.com

Mohan Debarchan Mohanty
College of Engineering and Technology, Bhubaneswar, India

Namrata P. Mohanty
Department of Computer Science & Engg, Siksha 'O' Anusandhan (Deemed to be University), Bhubaneswar, India. E-mail: namratam54@gmail.com

Saumendra Kumar Mohapatra
ITER, Siksha 'O' Anusandhan (Deemed to be University), Bhubaneswar, India

Sushree Bibhuprada B. Priyadarshini
Siksha 'O' Anusandhan (Deemed to be University), Bhubaneswar, India.
E-mail: bibhupradabimala@gmail.com

Amrit Sahani
Computer Science and Information Technology, Institute of Technical Education and Research, Siksha 'O' Anusandhan, (Deemed to be University), Bhubaneswar 751030, India.
E-mail: situnamrit@gmail.com

Sibani Sarangi
I.D.S, Siksha "O" Anusandhan, (Deemed to be University), Bhubaneswar, India

Devendra Kumar Sharma
Department of Electronics and Communication Engineering, IIMT Engineering College, SRM-IST, Ghaziabad, India. E-mail: d_k_s1970@yahoo.co.in

Debabrata Singh
ITER, Department of CSE, Siksha "O" Anusandhan, (Deemed to be University), Bhubaneswar, India. E-mail: debabratasingh@soa.ac.in

Tripti Swarnkar
Department of Computer Application, Siksha 'O' Anusandhan (Deemed to be University), Bhubaneswar, India. E-mail: triptiswarnakar@soa.ac.in

ABBREVIATIONS

AES	advanced encoding
ANN	artificial neural network
AOT	adenomatoid odontogenic tumor
BAN	body area network
BCI	brain-computer interface
BDA	big data analytics
BLE	Bluetooth low energy
BT	blended treatment
CDC	Centers for Disease Control and Prevention
CNN	Convolutional Neural Networks
CoAP	correspondence overhead influenced application protocol
CPS	cyber physical system
CSMA/CA	carrier sense multiple access—collision avoidance
CVD	cardiovascular disease
DBP	diastolic blood pressure
DDoS	distributed denial of service
DT	decision tree
ECC	elliptic curve steganography
ECG	electrocardiogram
EEG	electroencephalographic
EPC	electronic product code
FDT	fuzzy decision tree
GA	genetic algorithm
GUI	graphical user interface
HGG	high-grade glioma
Iaas	infrastructure as a service
IP	net protocol
IoMT	Internet of Medical Things
IoT	Internet of Things
KDD	Knowledge Discovery in Databases
LGG	low-grade glioma
LSTM	long short-term memory
MAC	media-get to controller

MB	megabytes
MF	membership function
MRF	random Markov field
MRI	magnetic resonance imaging
MS	multiple sclerosis
PACU	post-anesthesia care unit
PaaS	platform as a service
PB	petabytes
PKC	public-key steganography
PHY	physical circuits
RF	radio frequency
RF	random field
RFC	random forests classifier
RFID	radio frequency identification
SaaS	software as a service
SAM	selective attention mechanism
SBP	systolic blood pressure
SGF	Savitzky–Golay filter
SLIP	Serial Line Net Protocol
SOA	service-oriented architecture
TAU	treatment as usual
TCGA	threshold steganography-based bunch attestation
UVs	unmanned vehicles
WA	weighted average
WoT	Web of Things
WSN	wireless sensor networks

PREFACE

The current age of the Internet of Things (IoT) allures billions of users due to its wide range of popularity and broad range of applications in many fields of life. Modern technologies coupled with the Internet of Things (IoT) platform are evolving for patient care delivery.

In this text, we discuss how such novel technology affords a bridge for the development of the modern advanced healthcare system, incorporating patients as crucial actors in various ways, while decreasing costs and improving the treatment and diagnostics outcomes. IoT is basically an advanced automation and analytics framework in the context of biomedical that exploits networking, big data, sensing, and artificial intelligence technologies to deliver complete systems for either product or service. The advanced automation and analytics of IoT in medical applications allows more powerful emergency support services, which typically suffer from their limited resources.

In this connection, our book throws light on patient data gathering, elder care, as well as real-life location management, patient tracking through the usage of IoT technologies. Fundamentally, it collaborates regarding the IoT devices that are employed for enabling distant health tracking, emergency notification, etc. In addition to the fundamentals, it predominantly incorporates the cardiac problem analysis for e-healthcares while incorporating the concept of smart devices employed for different patients. Further, the analysis is elaborated while discussing its automation using Fuzzy Interference system. This book incorporates the use of smart wheelchairs, telemedicine, GPS positioning of heart patients, smart administration with drug tracking.

Again, it discusses the case studies that answers the issues related to enterprise/warehouse and responds to the anomaly pertaining to health in households for dependant persons. Furthermore, the analysis of heterogeneous data with large volume and diverse dimensionalities is elaborated. At length, the concept of regression and classification are discussed along with IoT applications in healthcare.

ORGANIZATION OF THE BOOK

The book is organized into eight chapters. A brief description of each of the chapters is as follows:

Chapter 1 focuses on the Internet of Things (IoT) in various uprights of the helpful business beginning from the drug watching and the administration to digitization of facilities with telemedicine care. This chapter examines every feasible region at which IoT advancement can be improved.

Chapter 2 targets information regarding the techniques for ECG analysis and IoT-based communication. Along with many techniques applied for analysis and diagnosis, the role of hybrid and optimized techniques are also incorporated.

Chapter 3 deals with various machine learning techniques applied for real-time data acquisition as well as classification for improved detection of depression from a early time. Moreover, the chapter illustrates the several IoT and machine learning work for helping the society for predicting depression as well as related seizures, trauma as well as injuries occurring within the brain.

Chapter 4 considers an extensive state-of-the-art survey on the role of decision tree in the context of soft computing, big data, while considering the IoT usage. In this context, various issues concerning the field of soft computing paradigms such as genetic algorithm, artificial neural network, and fuzzy logic have also been incorporated in this chapter.

Chapter 5 offers the working of IoT, its architecture and implementation in healthcare units like: electrocardiogram (ECG) monitoring, glucose level sensing, body temperature tracking, wheelchair handling, etc.

Chapter 6 comprehensively investigates various IoT technologies, their applications, and smart industrial management trends in IoT based on medical as well as healthcare solutions such that researchers will be able to highlight definite applications, statistics and products those get derived from healthcare pertaining to IoT domain.

Chapter 7 discusses regarding secured healthcare supervising system that adopts fuzzy logic-based decision platform, thus assisting in resolving the odontogenic tumors. Here, an aggregation of fuzzy logic as well as protected flexible model are employed in order to identify the status of the health patient.

Chapter 8 throws light on inaccessible patient perception framework under various conditions like: emergency clinics, home, etc. Various note worthy signs as well as therapeutic guide are maintained while considering IoT applications in healthcare.

KEY FEATURES OF THE BOOK

- Gives a lucid representation of the use of IoT in the field of biomedical engineering while exploring all the feasible forms of navigable information pertaining to biomedical engineering.
- Invariably refers to various current issues associated with biomedical engineering while including the fundamentals such as: collaboration on usage of sensors, bio-interfaces, telemedicine, remote healthcare, etc.
- Affords a platform that presents progress and research outcomes in the field of IoT in biomedical engineering that will bring together the ideas of scientists, researchers, and scholars in the domain of interest of the world.
- Highlights the current emerging features, lucid textual taxonomy while incorporating literary miscellanies and anthologies relevant to the field of biomedical aspects.
- Explores the integration of bio-interfaces, devices, sensors, techniques of telemedicine, etc. which make it a unique one.
- Throws light on Internet of Things for healthcare monitoring as well as remote healthcare, data communication, monitoring, and diagnosis.

CHAPTER 1

USE OF IoT IN BIOMEDICAL SIGNAL ANALYSIS FOR HEALTHCARE SYSTEMS

MIHIR NARAYAN MOHANTY[1*],
SAUMENDRA KUMAR MOHAPATRA[1], and
MOHAN DEBARCHAN MOHANTY[2]

[1]ITER, Siksha 'O' Anusandhan (Deemed to be University), Bhubaneswar, Odisha, India

[2]College of Engineering and Technology, Bhubaneswar, Odisha, India

*Corresponding author. E-mail: mihir.n.mohanty@gmail.com

ABSTRACT

Death rate is proportionally increasing with health ailment and accident throughout the world. Though technology develops day-by-day, still the gap is there in many areas. Especially the healthcare units lack to provide adequate support and solution to human society. Since last decade enormous developments have been done in technological field and applied in academia, industries, and healthcare units. Sophisticated analysis and diagnosis is still challenge for researchers that can help to the physicians as well to the society. In this chapter, authors focus on cardiac problem analysis for e-healthcares. For the data collection, smart sensors are used for different patients. Using the Arduino kit, the data can be transferred to cloud for internet-based uses. It will be easier to observe through either mobile devices or through computers. The analysis is automated using fuzzy inference system. Also it is developed for graphical user interface (GUI) to make the system user-friendly. The analysis and detection is performed well with the application of fuzzy logic. Due to such setup, communication can be bidirectional to diagnosis, monitoring, and suggestions. Some of the results are depicted in this scenario and some of the issues are kept as open challenges. Starting from individuals to data mining, many types of signals are analyzed and exhibited.

1.1 INTRODUCTION

Nowadays Internet of Things (IoT) is one of the buzzwords in information technology. The real-world objects can be transforms into intelligent and most effective objects by the application of IoT. It formulates an integrated communication atmosphere of interconnected devices and performs by engaging both the virtual and physical world together. Objects in remote areas can be controlled and accessed through IoT in an existing network structure. An opportunity can also be created for making a direct interaction between the physical world and computerized system. In 1982, the concept for creating a network of smart devices was designed by modifying a coke machine at Carnegie Mellon University and it became the first electrical device connected with the Internet.[1] IoT is a framework for the evaluating and monitoring of distributed data sources over a specified network environment. The idea of expanding the application of the Internet into real-world objects can be done by IoT. This trend is growing with positive impact worldwide and several industries are also adopting this technology to improve their service quality. The concept of IoT raised by the union of several advanced technologies such as machine learning, real-time data analysis, commodity sensors, and embedded systems. IoT system can be enabled by the contribution of the wireless sensor network, automation, embedded systems, and other advanced techniques.[2,3]

The IoT is a vibrant universal information network that consists of multiple objects that are connected through the Internet. These objects can be radio frequency identifiers, sensors, actuators, and other instruments and smart electrical devices. Over the last few decades, it can be observed that several small and medium enterprises and academic researchers are developing a huge amount of IoT solutions that can be applied in many industries such as e-commerce, healthcare sectors, agriculture, and waste management.[4] IoT plays an important role in healthcare sectors. Diagnosis system for several diseases can be integrated by applying IoT in hospitals. IoT-based healthcare system or also called smart healthcare system can be led to creating a digitalized patient service in remote areas. For the purpose of health monitoring and emergency notification, IoT devices can be enabled for monitoring the blood pressure and heart rate. Several advanced devices are there for monitoring some specific implants, such as pacemakers, Fitbit electronic wristbands, and hearing aids.[5] For detecting the patient's behaviors in bed, some hospitals are also started implementing the smart beds. By applying the IoT devices in the healthcare sector, the annual expenditure can be reduced and revenue can be increased in hospitals.[6,7] Different policies and guideline have been introduced for implementing IoT technology in the healthcare organizations in many countries. Still, this advanced technology remains in its infancy in the healthcare field.[15]

    The heart is the most vital organ of an individual. Its major function is to pump blood and distribute throughout the human organ. Cardiac disease is one of the top causes of death globally. The main factors behind cardiovascular disease (CVD) are high blood pressure, cholesterol, diet, alcohol consumption, etc. Electrocardiogram (ECG) system is a simple track of the electrical movements created by the heart. ECG is a powerful non-obtrusive instrument for different biomedical applications, for estimating the pulse, looking at the rhythm of pulses, diagnosing heart variations from the norm, emotion acknowledgment, and recognition of biometric proof.[8] With the innovations in embedded information and communication technologies, sophisticated healthcare support can be provided to human beings at any places. This technology can be useful for offering ECG monitoring facility to patients, senior citizens, athletes, and common people. By the use of this facility, the diagnosis of cardiac illness can be progressed with minimum time and expenditure.[9] ECG is detected by traditional large and stationary types of equipment in hospitals. To improve the diagnosis time, it is required to implement a smart low-cost ECG signal detection system that can transform data to hospitals from any places. In Figure 1.1, an IoT-based ECG data transmission system for the patients affected by CVD is presented. Due to the development in wireless sensor network, the transmission of ECG signals can be done easily to the hospitals through wireless transmission techniques such as Bluetooth or Zigbee.[10–12] In this system, the number of electrodes is less than traditional ECG data collecting system and can collect basic information of the heart. Long-term ECG signals can be monitored with minimal cost by this portable sensors. In Figure 1.2, the smart sensors equipment for ECG data recording is displayed.

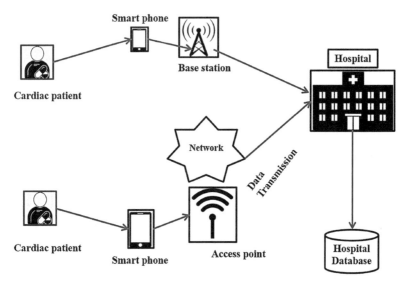

FIGURE 1.1 IoT-based ECG data transmission system.[10]

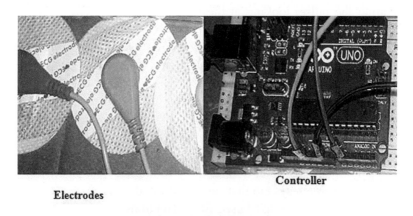

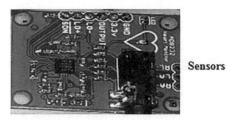

FIGURE 1.2 ECG data collection and monitoring equipment.[13]

In this chapter, a framework for IoT-based ECG data analysis system is proposed that can be deployed in any remote area for the diagnosis of cardiac diseases. Starting from the data collection to analysis and automatic disease detection, all are briefly discussed.

1.2 LITERATURE SURVEY

IoT is the concept of connecting anyone, anytime, anyplace, any service, and any network. It provides a particular solution for different applications such as smart cities, emergency services, traffic management, healthcare, logistic, and waste management.[14] Medicals and healthcare are one of the most effective application areas of IoT. It has the ability to improve healthcare services such as several disease diagnosis, remote health monitoring, patient management, and fitness programs. Researchers have given a wide range of attention for addressing the different applications of IoT in healthcare platform by considering multiple practical challenges. As a result of this, there are several applications, services, and prototypes of IoT in this field. IoT-based healthcare research includes architecture and platform of the network, new service, and applications, security, interoperability, and others. In the last few decades, a large number of works related to IoT-based healthcare system was addressed by the researchers. These include the smart treatment of different diseases such as cardiac illness, different chronic disease, and heartbeat monitor. Survey about the works related to this is discussed later.

In IoT-based ECG analysis, the data can be collected using wearable instruments, and for further analysis, it can be transmitted to cloud-based data storage system. This data transmission can be done by wireless data transmission method. Users can view the ECG data available at the cloud storage system by applying HTTP and MQTT protocols. This concept can take minimum time for the ECG analysis, and doctors can start the diagnosis at an early stage.[16] Analysis of biomedical signal by an IoT-based distributed framework was introduced for the monitoring of human physical activity. The body area network (BAN) was deployed in the human body to monitor the heart rate of a football player. The case study was applied during a football match, and the real-time data was collected to visualize the heart activity during the match. Some possible injuries were also detected by this system.[17] Continuous cardiac health monitoring is required in the case of the patients affected by heart diseases, and this can be done by enabling IoT-based ECG monitoring system. IoT-enabled ECG monitoring system can have different modules like signal sensing module, automatic signal quality assessment module, ECG analysis, and transmission modules. This overall system can also classify the ECG into acceptable and nonacceptable classes. It includes different electronics equipment like ECG sensors for data recording, Arduino board, Android mobile, Bluetooth, and cloud service for data storage. For validating the designed framework, some ECG signals were taken from MIT-BIH and Physionet databases. This IoT-enabled paradigm can be clinically accepted for improving the accuracy in automated diagnosis system.[18] A bridge is to be established between the doctors and the patients through which the communication can be done by the Internet for home care patients. This system was introduced for the treatment of some noncommunicable diseases.[19] IoT-based sensors can be installed in a patient's home for blood pressure measurement, ECG signal recording, a measure of sugar in the blood. Doctors can provide online treatment advice by analyzing these pathological data available at the web portal. For improving the healthcare monitoring in remote areas, the biomedical data collected by the sensors needs to transmit to the nearest gateway for advance processing. This data transmission process consumes a considerable amount of power and also the network traffic increases. To avoid these problems, a smart data transmission system was introduced that uses the IEEE 802.15.4 standard.[20] The power consumption and network traffic is quite minimum in event-based transmission system as compare to continuous transmission. Two different types of rule engines (static and dynamic) were developed for the ECG data transmission. The performance of the proposed model was measured by calculating the amount of power consumption and network traffic. Health monitoring can also be done by Android applications with IoT platform. Authors have designed an Android-based smart application "ECG Android App" for the visualization and transmission of ECG data to cloud storage.[21] These data stored at the cloud platform can be accessed by the expert physicians for the analysis of the behavior of the heart. It requires number of the equipment for developing such type of advanced medical application. The concept of fog computing–based patient monitoring system is an advanced framework in medical industries. This concept provides a smart platform that combines multiple technologies such as embedded data mining, distributed storage system, and notification service at the edge of the network.[22] Authors have chosen ECG signals as their case study and extracted useful features from the signal for the diagnosis of cardiac illness. From their result, it can be noticed that the bandwidth efficiency in fog computing concept is higher than 90%.

Besides ECG monitoring, also other diseases were monitored by using IoT-based smart healthcare. Human brain activity can be analyzed from electroencephalographic (EEG) changes. The driver's activity can be monitor through automatic analyzing his EEG signals for safe-driving purpose. A novel real-time wireless sensor–based EEG monitor system was developed to examine the driver's awareness activity.[23] That system was assembled with wireless and wearable EEG devices. They have validated the reliability of the proposed system with 15 participants. Noninvasive sensors are required for analyzing different human physiological parameters during the treatment. For this purpose, a wireless T-shirt was designed which is easy to wear and independent from the remote unit.[24] The data collected from this wearable sensorized T-shirt will be helpful for measuring different activities of the human body. For transmitting patient's physical activities to the medical applications in remote areas, a smart system was designed by the researchers.[25] That system can record the patient's blood pressure, ECG, peripheral capillary oxygen saturation, and some other factors. These data are transmitted over sample prototype to the hospital for doctor's analysis. Ultrasonic images play a major role for analysis of multiple diseases like obstetrics, abdominal, and cardiac illness. In rural areas, these images should be analyzed by the doctors to improve the treatment service. Different compression and transmission techniques for ultrasound images in remote were analyzed in Ref. [26]. An intelligent home care system was implemented to improve the home healthcare service.[27] That proposed platform is assembled with an intelligent medicine box with advanced connectivity. An improved service facility fuses IoT devices with in-home healthcare services. The in-home healthcare service includes the telemedicine facility. Two-stage medical data access and monitoring system were designed.[28] First a model is designed for storing and interrupting IoT data. After this, a data accessing method was configured for acquiring and processing of IoT data all over the place for improving the accessibility of IoT data sources. After this authors have presented an IoT-enabled device for emergency medical data collection and analysis. An Android-based platform was developed for measuring different parameters of the human being. That device can measure systolic blood pressure (SBP), diastolic blood pressure (DBP), and heart rate.

These data can be transmitted by using Bluetooth technique for comparing with standard range.[29] Different requirements for establishing smart high-level health services as the bridge (gateway) between the hospitals and the patients in the home are embedded data mining, storage system, smart data processing, etc. There are also many challenges for wireless smart data transmission system such as energy consumption, efficiency, reliability, and scalability of the system. IoT-based smart patient monitoring system that enhances these issues was proposed by the authors.[30]

1.2.1 IoT-BASED SMART DATA ACQUISITION AND PROCESSING SYSTEM

ECG is one of the important references for the diagnosis of many types of cardiac problem. Doctors can identify any disorder in the heart by visually analyzing the ECG recordings of the patients. Sometimes its acquisition directly affects the treatment of the cardiac patients. In traditional 12-lead ECG recording system, the electrodes are attached in different parts of the body as presented in Figure 1.3. The signal is recorded by a machine placed external to the human body. Generally, there are five major deflections in a cardiac signal that correspond to the amplitude, shape, location, and duration. These are generally called P, Q, R, S, and T waves. U wave is a small deflection in signal as displayed in Figure 1.4.

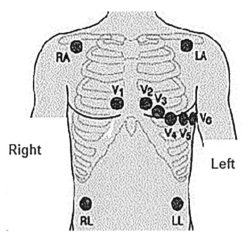

FIGURE 1.3 Electrode placement in the body during ECG recording in the traditional method.[47]

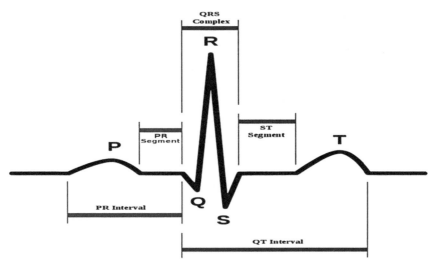

FIGURE 1.4 ECG signal with standard fiducial points.

The P wave corresponds to the atrial systole. This is a diminutive low-voltage deflection missing from the baseline. The P wave is related to the right and left atrial depolarization. Q wave is the starting element in the QRS complex, which is situated at the downward deflection after the P wave. R wave is another part of the QRS complex, which is first upward deflection after the P wave. S wave is the downward deflection after the R wave and is also a component in the QRS complex.[31] Q, R, and S waves are considered as QRS complex of the ECG signal, and this QRS feature is considered as the powerful feature for the ECG analysis. It represents the depolarization of both the left and right ventricular together. T wave represents the ventricular repolarization. Repolarization occurs on the opposite direction of the depolarization and it begins on the surface epicardium of the heart and it extends toward the endocardium. U wave typically follows the T wave on the ECG, and it is always typical in the direction of the T wave itself.[32] QRS complex feature is one of the most used features for ECG signal analysis.

These traditional types of equipment are not portable, and sometimes these systems are not suitable for analyzing the long duration ECG of a patient. They can't be used at the home due to their expense, and patients have to visit hospitals repeatedly, and the burden increases for both hospitals and patients' attendants. To overcome this problem, a portable long-term

ECG recording machine is highly required that can easily record human's cardiac function with minimum time, and data can be transmitted to the hospitals.[33] A framework for smart ECG system is presented in Figure 1.5.[13] Other devices can be deployed for measuring different parameters of the human body such as heartbeat measuring sensors, pulse rate, and devices for measuring SpO2 as an alternative. These portable devices can be used for home care patients. Doctors can also verify and analyze these data without patient visits hospitals. Different smart devices for measuring this parameter are presented in Figures 1.6 and 1.7. In heartbeat measuring sensors, the amount of blood flowing to the fingers with respect to time can be recorded. For calculating the heart rate, a sensor is assembled with LM358 OP-AMP that monitors the heartbeat pulses.

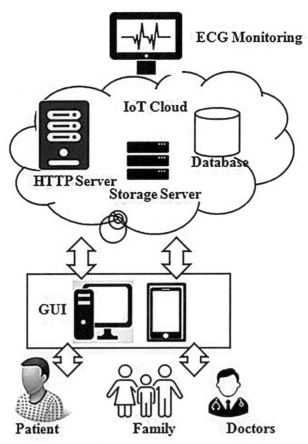

FIGURE 1.5 IoT-based automatic ECG monitoring system.[13]

Use of IoT in Biomedical Signal Analysis   11

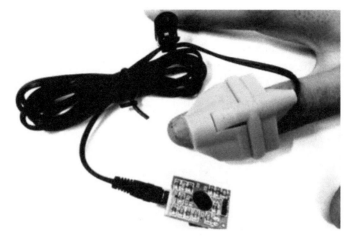

FIGURE 1.6 A smart device for measuring heartbeat.

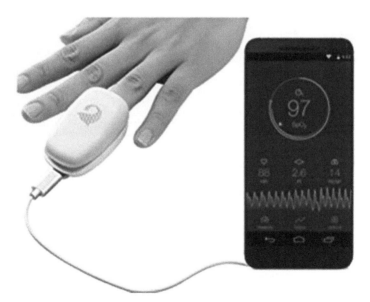

FIGURE 1.7 Smart SpO2 measuring device.

1.3 IoT-BASED COMMUNICATION

It is another important task to monitor and analyze the data collected by smart devices. Several sensors and other instruments are required for this advanced healthcare system. These devices may be some specialized device or smartphones. Data transmission can be performed by applying the BAN concept.[34] Arduino-based ECG data recording machine is proposed, which is monitored by a portable computer. ECG data is collected from the patients and is sent to cloud. The overall process is performed using Arduino board. It will helpful for mobile devices as well. Figure 1.8 is the setup for communication system, and the corresponding output is shown in Figure 1.9.

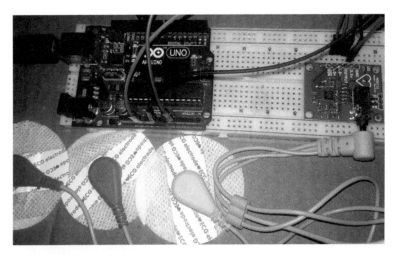

FIGURE 1.8   Arduino setup for ECG recording.

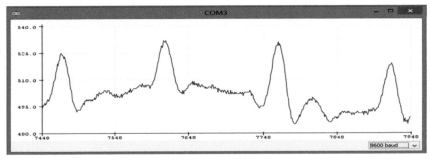

FIGURE 1.9   ECG signals recorded by Arduino setup.

In our proposed work, we have also considered an open-source database for validation purpose. In Table 1.1, a detailed ECG data source is presented. MIT-BIH Arrhythmia Database is chosen for the validation of the result. A sample Arrhythmia ECG plot is shown in Figure 1.10.

TABLE 1.1 Different ECG Database.

Databases	Samples	Sampling frequency (Hz)
MIT-BIH arrhythmia	48	360
MIT-BIH normal sinus rhythm	18	128
Noise stress test	12 ECG 3 Noise	360
Atrial fibrillation	25	250
T-wave alternans	100	500
Supraventricular arrhythmia	78	128
Malignant ventricular arrhythmia	22	250
Long-term database	7	128
MIT-BIH-ST change	28	360
PTB	549	1000
QT	105	250
Apnea-ECG	70	100
Non-invasive fetal ECG	55	1000
Creighton University ventricular tachyarrhythmia database	35	250
American Heart Association database short/long	10/67	250
Fantasia	40	250
BIDMC congestive heart failure	15	250
European ST-T	90	250
Long-term ST	86	250
IN-CART	75	257

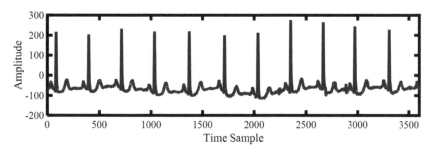

FIGURE 1.10 MIT-BIH arrhythmia ECG.

1.3.1 NOISE REMOVAL FROM THE ECG SIGNAL

Most of the ECG signals are noisy in nature because those are infected by several varieties of noise. It happens due to many factors like cable connections, variations in the electrode impedances, and movement of the patients.[35] Removal of this unwanted particle from this cardiac signal is the most important job for the purpose of accurate diagnosis. The goal of the preprocessing stage is to decrease the noise level and avoid waveform distortion.[36] Generally, there are two types of noises that influence ECG. Baseline wander noise is a nonstationary sinusoidal signal, and it happens due to the outcome of baseline drift. It can be measured as an amplitude inflection to the ECG. Power line interference is another type of noise that often appears in the ECG signal. This interference can be caused by electromagnetic interference by a power line, electromagnetic field by the machinery if it is placed nearby, improper grounding of ECG machine or patients.[37,38] Besides these types of noise, there are some other disturbances affecting the signal. These are as follows:

  I. Electrode contact noise: It happens due to the deficit in the contiguity among the electrode and skin.
  II. Electrode motion artifacts: Artifacts that comes from deviations in the electrode–skin impedance with electrode motion.
  III. Muscle contractions (electromyography noise): It is the type of noise that comes from the contraction of other muscles other than the heart.
  IV. Instrumentation noise: This type of noise is generally produced from the electronic equipment used for ECG recording.
  V. Electrosurgical noise: Medical equipment noises at frequencies between 100 kHz and 1 MHz

Physicians face difficulty for the diagnosis of a cardiac patient because of this unwanted particle in the ECG. Therefore, denoising of ECG signal and preprocessing is an important task in CVD classification. Therefore, there are different types of preprocessing steps for a better classification of cardiac disease.[39]

Filtering is the initial state in preprocessing of the ECG. In this stage, different types of filtering blocks are used for removing the unwanted elements from the signal. Finite impulse response (FIR) and infinite impulse response are two different types of filters that can be applied in order to denoising the ECG signal.[40] FIR filters are treated as a non-recursive digital filter that is used for the cleaning purpose of the ECG signal. This filter decreases most of the noises in the frequency range of 0–100 Hz, and this frequency level may increase based on the design of the filter.[41] There are several types of filters that were used by the researchers in order to obtain a clean ECG for good analysis and classification. Band-pass filter, high-pass filter, and Savitzky–Golay filter (SGF) are the most used filters for ECG noise removal.[42,43]

Here the denoising of the raw ECG signals is done by applying a SGF. For the smoothening purpose of data points, this type of filter can be considered. It will help to increase the SNR without affecting the original signal. By applying the linear least square method, low-degree polynomial data points are created for discarding the noise particle from the signal. The convolutional coefficients can be found by equally separating the data points. For archiving the smoothed signal, these convolutional coefficients will be applied at the central points of each data points. The observed smooth signal is represented by the following equation:

$$Y_k = \sum C_i y_{k+i}, \frac{m-1}{2} \leq k \leq n - \frac{m-1}{2} \qquad (1.1)$$

where C_i is the filter and n is the length of the signal. m is the order of the filter for m point quadratic polynomial. Y_k is the observed smoothed signal. y is the sample data, $k = 1,\ldots, n$.[44]

1.3.2 FUZZY LOGIC–BASED DISEASE DETECTION SYSTEM

Healthcare research suggests that cardiac abnormality begins with damage to the inner layers of heart arteries. The following factors may create damage:

    i.   If the blood pressure is high
   ii.   If the cholesterol is high
  iii.   If the blood sugar is high
  iv.   If blood vessel inflammation occurs.

Nowadays, coronary heart disease is the most common form of CVD. Different related tests may be undertaken in order to make an accurate diagnosis. Usually, physicians prescribe the following minimal tests for any cardiac patients.

- A blood test to know the levels of various factors such as electrolytes, blood cells, hormones in the blood, and clotting factors. Also, the sugar level in blood can be verified.
- ECG may show changes that indicate the heart muscle is not receiving enough oxygen.

For automatic detecting any cardiac problem, a system is introduced based on fuzzy logic. It can detect whether the patient has any cardiac disorder or not. The detailed information about the proposed interface is presented in the following sections.

1.3.3 FUZZY RULES AND FUZZY SYSTEM

The implementation of fuzzy logic to the real-world problems is appropriate as these problems are imprecise rather than exact. The behavior of the human brain is assumed as a combination of fuzzy concepts, fuzzy judgments, and fuzzy reasoning. Again fuzzy logic deals with natural language, and the problem domain is easily described in linguistic terms. Fuzzy classification techniques provide soft decision rather than a hard decision.

The fuzzy set is defined without a hard boundary and degree of the membership of an element can be expressed with a real number in the range 0–1.

S is a fuzzy set on U that defines an ordered pair $(a, \mu B(a))$ such that:

$$S = \{a, \mu B(a)\, a, 0 \leq \mu B(a) \leq 1\} \tag{1.2}$$

Here $\mu B(a)$ is the membership function (MF) of each a in S, and it shows membership degree concept for an element a to a set S and $\mu B(a) \in [0; 1]$.

1.3.4 STEPS INVOLVED IN THE FUZZY INFERENCE SYSTEM

Fuzzification—The conversion of the collected data to a set of suitable fuzzy variables is called fuzzification. This is the first step in fuzzy logic in which values to each MF are given. The MF take various shapes such as triangular, trapezoidal, and Gaussian. For the modeling of the system, triangular and trapezoidal MF[45,46] are used and are explained as follows.

1.3.5 TRIANGULAR MEMBERSHIP FUNCTION

Let $\{o, p, q\}$ is the set of parameters

Triangle $(y; o, p, q) = 0$ if $y \leq o$;
or $= (y-o)(p-o)$ if $o \leq y \leq p$;
or $= (y-p)(q-p)$ if $p \leq y \leq q$;
or $= 0$ if $q \geq y$.

1.3.6 TRAPEZOIDAL MEMBERSHIP FUNCTION

Let $\{o, p, q, r\}$ is the set of parameters

Trapezoidal $(y; o, p, q, r) = 0$ if $y \leq o$;
or $= (y-o)(p-o)$ if $o \leq y \leq p$;
or $= 1$ if $p \leq y \leq q$;
or $= (r-y)(r-q)$ if $q \leq y \leq r$;
(3) or $= 0$ if $y \geq r$.

1.3.7 FUZZY RULE

The system operates on rules that are in the form of IF…THEN or IF…THEN…ELSE. The antecedents of the rule are taken with IF and the consequent part comes after THEN. The linguistic variables are converted into rules taking the fuzzy values, that is, the words representing the fuzzy terms are converted into a fuzzy subset of a particular problem. There are many variants of fuzzy rules out of which we have taken Sugeno or Takagi–Sugeno rules. Though fuzzification of inputs and use of fuzzy operators are the same for both Mamdani and Sugeno method, there is a difference in the output of MF. The output of the Sugeno method is either linear or constant. For a Sugeno fuzzy model having inputs x and y and the output z, o, p, and q are taken as constants. Output for the Sugeno-based model is numerical.

1.3.8 FUZZY INFERENCE SYSTEM

The four parameters that are considered for the diagnosis are fuzzified as follows:

ECG—Three types of fuzzy sets such as ST-T, abnormal, and hypertrophy are considered for the defuzzification of ECG. The trapezoidal MF is considered for normal and hypertrophies fuzzy set. For ST-T fuzzy set, triangular MF is chosen.

Blood pressure—Detailed parameters for blood pressure are presented in Table 1.2. In our proposed approach, SBP is considered.

TABLE 1.2 Fuzzy Set Details for Blood Pressure.

Fuzzy set	Membership function
Low	Trapezoidal
Normal	Triangular
High	Trapezoidal

MF and fuzzy set details for fasting blood sugar and cholesterol are presented in Tables 1.3 and 1.4. Figures 1.11–1.14 show MF for input data.

TABLE 1.3 Fuzzy Set Details for Blood Sugar.

Fuzzy set	Membership function
Low (<10)	Trapezoidal
Normal (70–135)	Triangular
High (>130)	Trapezoidal

TABLE 1.4 Fuzzy Set Details for Blood Cholesterol.

Fuzzy set	Membership function
Less risk (200)	Trapezoidal
Borderline high (190–245)	Triangular
High (240)	Trapezoidal

1.4 FUZZY KNOWLEDGE REPRESENTATION

The decision **D** will be taken by the system for a certain disease by analyzing values of the fuzzy set. Each value specifies the features of a disease. Three sets are considered in our work such as YES, MAYBE, and NO. The detailed structure of the fuzzy set is shown in Figure 1.15.

Use of IoT in Biomedical Signal Analysis 19

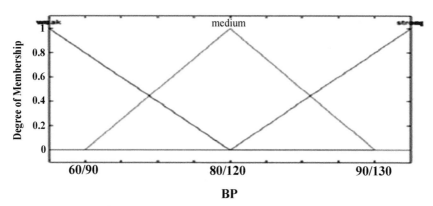

FIGURE 1.11 MF for blood pressure.

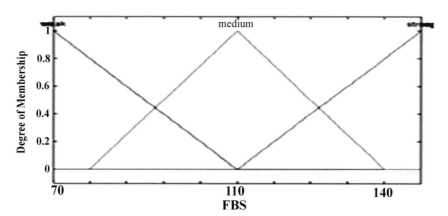

FIGURE 1.12 MF for fasting blood sugar.

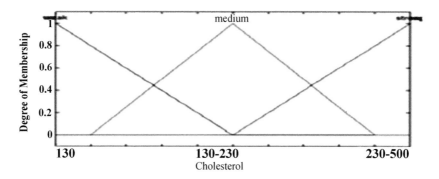

FIGURE 1.13 MF for fasting cholesterol.

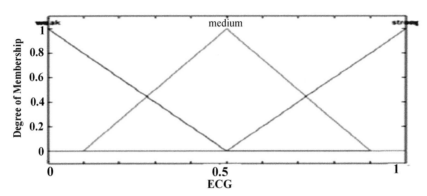

FIGURE 1.14 MF for fasting ECG.

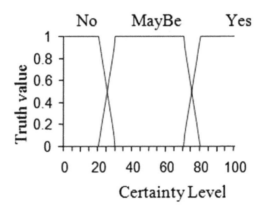

FIGURE 1.15 Fuzzy set for the diseases present in human body.

For a particular disease, there are some relevant features and these are the subsets of the collected feature set. A physician suggests some appropriate values for each entry of the disease profile. This work is done for each considered disease.

1.4.1 ALGORITHM

10 inputs: age, gender, chest pain type, cholesterol, blood pressure, fasting blood sugar, heart beat, ECG, exercise, heart disease category.
Output: Condition of heart disease is shown is linguistic terms.
Fuzzy variables are in each input.

The MF is assigned and calculated for each fuzzy variable.
Strength of the fuzzy rule is measured from the MF.
Category of the heart disease is determined from the maximum selected outputs.

Different MF for each input and output are presented in Figures 1.16–1.19. Figure 1.20 shows the input FIS editor.

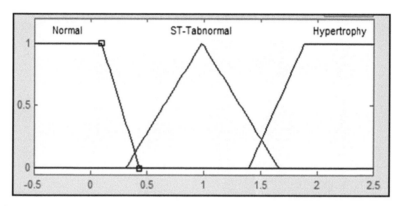

FIGURE 1.16 ECG MF.

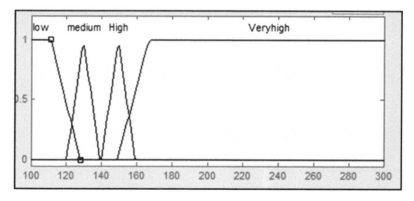

FIGURE 1.17 Blood pressure MF.

1.4.2 DEFUZZIFICATION

In the defuzzification process, obtained output variables are converted to real values. These values are useful for knowing the system information and can be useful for taking any action. Generally, two types of defuzzification methods are there in Sugeno model. They are weighted average (WA) and weighted sum. WA defuzzification method is considered in the proposed work.

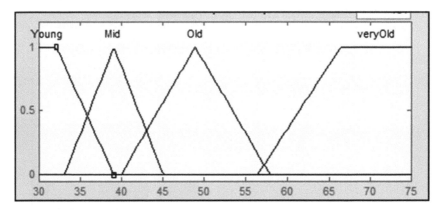

FIGURE 1.18 Age MF.

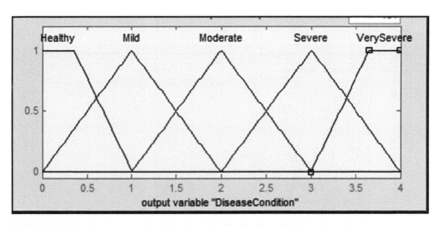

FIGURE 1.19 Output membership function for fasting cholesterol as input.

1.4.3 FUZZY INFERENCE

After proper diagnosis, the symptom S would be will be obtained. S is a natural value that specifies the strength of the nonmeasurable feature by a fuzzy variable. Besides this, there are also some other measurable features

Use of IoT in Biomedical Signal Analysis

such as temperature, pressure, and blood sugar, and these are specified some specific numbers.

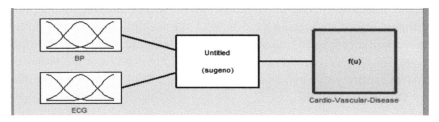

FIGURE 1.20 Inputs and outputs in FIS editor window.

1.5 RESULTS AND DISCUSSION

The accessed data is represented in Table 1.5. From the data, it can be observed that the patient is suffering from cardiac diseases. A snapshot for the data accessed in the MATLAB environment is presented in Figure 1.21.

TABLE 1.5 Obtained Data from the Patient.

Blood pressure	Cholesterol	Fasting blood sugar
97/165	480	270
98/150	450	180

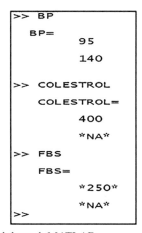

FIGURE 1.21 Data accessed through MATLAB.

The earlier-proposed fuzzy model is considered for the validation purpose. Information setup is one of the measure challenges in this system. For communicating the exact result, accurate test result is to coordinate. This agent-based e-healthcare system will be suitable for adopting different information about the disease. Here multiple agents are assigned to work in a combined manner. It is also adopting less time for detection of any disease. Some snapshots of the result obtained from the proposed system are presented in the latter figures. Figure 1.22 shows the input data for the system with MF.

PID	Age	YoungMF	MidMF	OldMF	VeryOldMF
2	63	0	0	0	1
3	67	0	0	0	1
4	67	0	0	0	1
5	37	0.11	0.8	0	0
6	41	0	0.57	0.13	0
7	56	0	0	0.2	0.5
8	62	0	0	0	1
9	57	0	0	0.1	0.63

FIGURE 1.22 Input data with MF.

For validation of the proposed system, the ECG data are chosen from the MIT-BIH arrhythmia database. It contains the data of the patient suffering from the arrhythmia, and a good result has been achieved. The diagnosis report and fuzzy graphical user interface (GUI) are presented in Figures 1.23 and 1.24.

1.6 CONCLUSION

This chapter provides information regarding the techniques for ECG analysis and IoT-based communication. Though many techniques are applied for analysis and diagnosis, still the researchers can work for hybrid and optimized techniques. Only a few works have been done in this area. To facilitate the patients and physicians of remote area, the communication techniques should be well developed. Similarly the way of communication can enhance for seamless services. The techniques of communication can be user-friendly so that everyone can use them.

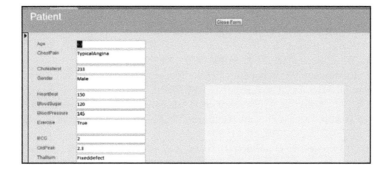

Age	Gender	Chest pain	Cholestreol	Heart beat	Blood Sugar	BloodPressure	Exercise	ECG	Oldpeak	Tinallum	HeartDisease
37	Male	Aypical Angina	250	187	90	130	FALSE	0	3.5	Normal	Severe
47	Male	Aypical Angina	204	172	100	130	TRUE	2	1.4	Normal	Severe
56	Male	Nonangina	236	178	100	120	FALSE	0	0.8	Normal	Severe
62	Female	Nonangina	268	160	90	140	FALSE	2	3.6	Normal	Severe
57	Female	Asymptomatic	354	163	100	120	TRUE	0	0.6	Normal	VerySevere
63	Male	Asymptomatic	254	147	110	130	FALSE	2	1.4	ReversibleDef	VerySevere
53	Male	Asymptomatic	203	155	106	140	TRUE	2	3.1	ReversibleDef	VerySevere
56	Male	Nonangina	256	142	100	130	TRUE	2	0.6	FixedDef	Severe
44	Male	Aypical Angina	263	173	100	120	FALSE	0	0	ReversibleDef	Mild

FIGURE 1.23 Diagnosis report for heart disease.

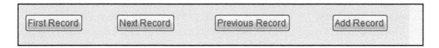

FIGURE 1.24 Input GUI for fuzzy interference system.

KEYWORDS

- **smart healthcare system**
- **cardiac disease**
- **IoT**
- **ECG**
- **e-healthcare**

REFERENCES

1. Gokhale, P.; Bhat, O.; Bhat, S. Introduction to IOT. *Int. J. Adv. Sci. Eng. Inf. Technol.* **2018,** *5*(1), 41–44.
2. Mattern, F.; Floerkemeier, C. From the Internet of Computers to the Internet of Things. In *From Active Data Management to Event-Based Systems and More*; Springer: Berlin, Heidelberg, 2010; pp 242–259.
3. AbuMansour, H. Y.; Elayyan, H. IoT Theme for Smart Datamining-Based Environment to Unify Distributed Learning Management Systems. In *2018 9th International Conference on Information and Communication Systems (ICICS)*; IEEE, April 2018; pp 212–217.
4. Mohanta, B.; Patnaik, S.; Patnaik, S. Big Data for Modelling Interactive Systems in IoT. In *2018 2nd International Conference on Data Science and Business Analytics (ICDSBA)*; IEEE, September 2018; pp 105–110.
5. Ersue, M.; Romascanu, D.; Schoenwaelder, J.; Sehgal, A. Management of Networks with Constrained Devices: Use Cases (No. RFC 7548), 2015.
6. da Costa, C. A.; Pasluosta, C. F.; Eskofier, B.; da Silva, D. B.; da Rosa Righi, R. Internet of Health Things: Toward Intelligent Vital Signs Monitoring in Hospital Wards. *Artif. Intell. Med.* **2018,** *89*, 61–69.
7. Roman, D. H.; Conlee, K. D.; Abbott, I.; Jones, R. P.; Noble, A.; Rich, N.; ... Costa, D. *The Digital Revolution Comes to US Healthcare*; Goldman Sachs: New York, NY, 2015.
8. Mohapatra, S. K.; Mohanty, M. N. ECG Analysis: A Brief Review. *Recent Pat. Comput. Sci.* **2019,** *12*, 1. https://doi.org/10.2174/2213275912666190408111123.
9. Mohammed, J.; Lung, C. H.; Ocneanu, A.; Thakral, A.; Jones, C.; Adler, A. Internet of Things: Remote Patient Monitoring Using Web Services and Cloud Computing. In *2014 IEEE International Conference on Internet of Things (iThings), and IEEE Green Computing and Communications (GreenCom) and IEEE Cyber, Physical and Social Computing (CPSCom)*; IEEE, September 2014; pp 256–263.
10. Neyja, M.; Mumtaz, S.; Huq, K. M. S.; Busari, S. A.; Rodriguez, J.; Zhou, Z. An IoT-Based E-Health Monitoring System Using ECG Signal. In *GLOBECOM 2017 – 2017 IEEE Global Communications Conference*; IEEE, December 2017; pp 1–6.
11. Xiong, X.; Zheng, K.; Xu, R.; Xiang, W.; Chatzimisios, P. Low Power Wide Area Machine-to-Machine Networks: Key Techniques and Prototype. *IEEE Commun. Mag.* **2015,** *53* (9), 64–71.
12. Lei, L.; Kuang, Y.; Cheng, N.; Shen, X. S.; Zhong, Z.; Lin, C. Delay-Optimal Dynamic Mode Selection and Resource Allocation in Device-to-Device Communications—Part I: Optimal Policy. *IEEE Trans. Veh. Technol.* **2015,** *65* (5), 3474–3490.
13. Yang, Z.; Zhou, Q.; Lei, L.; Zheng, K.; Xiang, W. An IoT-Cloud Based Wearable ECG Monitoring System for Smart Healthcare. *J. Med. Syst.* **2016,** *40* (12), 286.
14. Islam, S. R.; Kwak, D.; Kabir, M. H.; Hossain, M.; Kwak, K. S. The Internet of Things for Healthcare: A Comprehensive Survey. *IEEE Access* **2015,** *3*, 678–708.
15. Catarinucci, L.; De Donno, D.; Mainetti, L.; Palano, L.; Patrono, L.; Stefanizzi, M. L.; Tarricone, L. An IoT-Aware Architecture for Smart Healthcare Systems. *IEEE IoT J.* **2015,** *2* (6), 515–526.

16. Yang, Z.; Zhou, Q.; Lei, L.; Zheng, K.; Xiang, W. An IoT-Cloud Based Wearable ECG Monitoring System for Smart Healthcare. *J. Med. Syst.* **2016**, *40* (12), 286.
17. Mora, H.; Gil, D.; Terol, R. M.; Azorín, J.; Szymanski, J. An IoT-Based Computational Framework for Healthcare Monitoring in Mobile Environments. *Sensors* **2017**, *17* (10), 2302.
18. Satija, U.; Ramkumar, B.; Manikandan, M. S. Real-Time Signal Quality-Aware ECG Telemetry System for IoT-Based Healthcare Monitoring. *IEEE IoT J.* **2017**, *4* (3), 815–823.
19. Liu, Y.; Niu, J.; Yang, L.; Shu, L. eBPlatform: An IoT-Based System for NCD Patients Homecare in China. In *2014 IEEE Global Communications Conference*; IEEE, December 2014; pp 2448–2453.
20. Kiran, M. S.; Rajalakshmi, P.; Bharadwaj, K.; Acharyya, A. Adaptive Rule Engine Based IoT Enabled Remote Healthcare Data Acquisition and Smart Transmission System. In *2014 IEEE World Forum on Internet of Things (WF-IoT)*; IEEE, March 2014; pp 253–258.
21. Mohammed, J.; Lung, C. H.; Ocneanu, A.; Thakral, A.; Jones, C.; Adler, A. Internet of Things: Remote Patient Monitoring Using Web Services and Cloud Computing. In *2014 IEEE International Conference on Internet of Things (iThings), and IEEE Green Computing and Communications (GreenCom) and IEEE Cyber, Physical and Social Computing (CPSCom)*; IEEE, September 2014; pp 256–263.
22. Gia, T. N.; Jiang, M.; Rahmani, A. M.; Westerlund, T.; Liljeberg, P.; Tenhunen, H. Fog Computing in Healthcare Internet of Things: A Case Study on ECG Feature Extraction. In *2015 IEEE International Conference on Computer and Information Technology; Ubiquitous Computing and Communications; Dependable, Autonomic and Secure Computing; Pervasive Intelligence and Computing*; IEEE, October 2015; pp 356–363.
23. Lin, C. T.; Chuang, C. H.; Huang, C. S.; Tsai, S. F.; Lu, S. W.; Chen, Y. H.; Ko, L. W. Wireless and Wearable EEG System for Evaluating Driver Vigilance. *IEEE Trans. Biomed. Circuits Syst.* **2014**, *8* (2), 165–176.
24. Sardini, E.; Serpelloni, M.; Pasqui, V. Wireless Wearable T-Shirt for Posture Monitoring During Rehabilitation Exercises. *IEEE Trans. Instrum. Meas.* **2014**, *64* (2), 439–448.
25. Li, C.; Hu, X.; Zhang, L. The IoT-Based Heart Disease Monitoring System for Pervasive Healthcare Service. *Procedia Comput. Sci.* **2017**, *112*, 2328–2334.
26. Akkala, V.; Bharath, R.; Rajalakshmi, P.; Kumar, P. Compression Techniques for IoT Enabled Handheld Ultrasound Imaging System. In *2014 IEEE Conference on Biomedical Engineering and Sciences (IECBES)*; IEEE, December 2014; pp 648–652.
27. Yang, G.; Xie, L.; Mäntysalo, M.; Zhou, X.; Pang, Z.; Da Xu, L.; … Zheng, L. R. A Health-IoT Platform Based on the Integration of Intelligent Packaging, Unobtrusive Bio-Sensor, and Intelligent Medicine Box. *IEEE Trans. Ind. Inf.* **2014**, *10* (4), 2180–2191.
28. Xu, B.; Da Xu, L.; Cai, H.; Xie, C.; Hu, J.; Bu, F. Ubiquitous Data Accessing Method in IoT-Based Information System for Emergency Medical Services. *IEEE Trans. Ind. Inf.* **2014**, *10* (2), 1578–1586.
29. Antonovici, D. A.; Chiuchisan, I.; Geman, O.; Tomegea, A. Acquisition and Management of Biomedical Data Using Internet of Things Concepts. In *2014 International*

Symposium on Fundamentals of Electrical Engineering (ISFEE); IEEE, November 2014; pp 1–4.
30. Rahmani, A. M.; Thanigaivelan, N. K.; Gia, T. N.; Granados, J.; Negash, B.; Liljeberg, P.; Tenhunen, H. Smart E-Health Gateway: Bringing Intelligence to Internet-of-Things Based Ubiquitous Healthcare Systems. In *2015 12th Annual IEEE Consumer Communications and Networking Conference (CCNC)*; IEEE, January 2015; pp 826–834.
31. Karimipour, A.; Homaeinezhad, M. R. Real-Time Electrocardiogram P-QRS-T Detection–Delineation Algorithm Based on Quality-Supported Analysis of Characteristic Templates. *Comput. Biol. Med.* **2014,** *52*, 153–165.
32. Bognár, G.; Fridli, S. Heartbeat Classification of ECG Signals Using Rational Function Systems. In *International Conference on Computer Aided Systems Theory*; Springer, Cham, February 2017; pp 187–195.
33. Baig, M. M.; Gholamhosseini, H. Smart Health Monitoring Systems: An Overview of Design and Modeling. *J. Med. Syst.* **2013,** *37*(2), 9898.
34. Dhar, S. K.; Bhunia, S. S.; Mukherjee, N. Interference Aware Scheduling of Sensors in IoT Enabled Healthcare Monitoring System. In *2014 Fourth International Conference of Emerging Applications of Information Technology*; IEEE, December 2014; pp 152–157.
35. Duskalov, I. K.; Dotsinsky, I. A.; Christov, I. I. Developments in ECG Acquisition, Preprocessing, Parameter Measurement, and Recording. *IEEE Eng. Med. Biol. Mag.* **1998,** *17* (2), 50–58.
36. Agante, P. M.; De Sá, J. M. ECG Noise Filtering Using Wavelets with Soft-Thresholding Methods. In *Computers in Cardiology*; IEEE, 1999; pp 535–538.
37. Poungponsri, S.; Yu, X. H. An Adaptive Filtering Approach for Electrocardiogram (ECG) Signal Noise Reduction Using Neural Networks. *Neurocomputing* **2013,** *117*, 206–213.
38. Kapil, S.; Chawla, M.; Ansari, M. D. On K-Means Data Clustering Algorithm with Genetic Algorithm. In *2016 Fourth International Conference on Parallel, Distributed and Grid Computing (PDGC)*; IEEE, December 2016; pp 202–206.
39. Awal, M. A.; Mostafa, S. S.; Ahmad, M.; Rashid, M. A. An Adaptive Level Dependent Wavelet Thresholding for ECG Denoising. *Biocybern. Biomed. Eng.* **2014,** *34* (4), 238–249.
40. Mugdha, A. C.; Rawnaque, F. S.; Ahmed, M. U. A Study of Recursive Least Squares (RLS) Adaptive Filter Algorithm in Noise Removal from ECG Signals. In *Informatics, Electronics & Vision (ICIEV), 2015 International Conference on*; IEEE, June 2015; pp 1–6.
41. Patro, K. K.; Kumar, P. R. De-noising of ECG Raw Signal by Cascaded Window Based Digital Filters Configuration. In *Power, Communication and Information Technology Conference (PCITC)*; IEEE, October 2015; pp 120–124.
42. Javadi, M.; Arani, S. A. A. A.; Sajedin, A.; Ebrahimpour, R. Classification of ECG Arrhythmia by a Modular Neural Network Based on Mixture of Experts and Negatively Correlated Learning. *Biomed. Signal Process. Control* **2013,** *8* (3), 289–296.
43. Ebrahimpour, R.; Sadeghnejad, N.; Sajedin, A.; Mohammadi, N. Electrocardiogram Beat Classification via Coupled Boosting by Filtering and Preloaded Mixture of Experts. *Neural Comput. Appl.* **2013,** *23* (3–4), 1169–1178.

44. Mohanty, M. N. Denoising of ECG Signal Using Savitzky-Golay Filter. *J. Commun. Eng. Syst.* **2018,** *8* (2), 98–104.
45. Devi, C. S.; Ramani, G. G.; Pandian, J. A. Intelligent E-healthcare Management System in Medicinal Science. *Int. J. PharmTech Res* **2014,** *6* (6), 1838–1845.
46. Hussain, A.; Wenbi, R.; Xiaosong, Z.; Hongyang, W.; da Silva, A. L. Personal Home Healthcare System for the Cardiac Patient of Smart City Using Fuzzy Logic. *J. Adv. Inf. Technol.* **2016,** *7* (1).
47. https://mungfali.com/explore.php?q=Telemetry%20Lead%20Placement%20Di%E2%80%A6.

CHAPTER 2

APPLICATION OF THE INTERNET OF THINGS (IoT) FOR BIOMEDICAL PEREGRINATION AND SMART HEALTHCARE

ARADHANA BEHURA[1] and
SUSHREE BIBHUPRADA B. PRIYADARSHINI[2*]

[1]*Veer Surendra Sai University of Technology, Burla, Odisha, India*

[2]*Siksha 'O' Anusandhan Deemed to be University, Bhubaneswar, Odisha, India*

*Corresponding author. E-mail: bibhupradabimala@gmail.com

ABSTRACT

Interfacing the world with innovations has made a huge difference. Applications of the Internet of things (IoT) have been utilized in biomedical framework; however, the IoT has been larger than simply adding the network to the current items and administrations such that the items have moved toward becoming administrations themselves, and these have turned out to be progressively shrewd. Furthermore, telemedicine requires the fast, protected, enduring, and versatile arrangement of correspondence, so as to accomplish the point in which the specialists and patients can communicate continuously. In the future, IoT will drive another period of the medicine, and the hospitalization technique for the patients will likewise have a progressive change. Intelligent meeting represents a live discussion that utilizes proficient video conferencing frameworks for remote medicinal specialists and doctors as well as patients "up close and personal." In this connection, nonintuitive counsel is a nonlive interview through which the specialists concentrate the review information and other data of the patients exchanged through the system. It consolidates answers for the utilization of telemedicine and would altogether be able to lessen the time and cost of transporting patients.

Moreover, many specialists can break the point of confinement of the geographical degree, while sharing the case history and diagnostic. In general, enormous extending telemedicine applications can incredibly decrease the boundaries to patients accepting therapeutic consideration on the grounds that land segregation is never again a restorative unfavorable obstruction. This has incorporated segments, procedures, and security such as fighting against pharmaceutical problem and counterfeit items that identify with the restorative utilization of an IoT framework. By applying IoT, we can make smart chair that is helpful for blind people and work on information security, node mobility management in large-scale network, and many real-time problems such as kidnapping of newborn babies, and by applying global positioning system (GPS), we will be able to be aware about many diseases such as heart and brain tumors. The chapter discusses about the executed framework and how it functions with the assistance of test system and equipment stages. It answers a few issues related with IoT and shows how they work in the actualized framework in distinctive stages. The outcomes demonstrate the framework capacities easily on both test system condition and equipment stages, having the ability to be executed in an emergency clinic condition. Beginning from the medication observation and the execution to digitization of clinics and telemedicine care, we discussed each conceivable zone in which IoT innovation can upgrade the procedures.

2.1 INTRODUCTION

In human services space, wireless body area network has happened as a noticeable innovation that is equipped for giving better strategies for ongoing patient well-being checking at medical clinics, refuges, and even at their homes. As of late, WBAN (wireless body area network) has increased incredible intrigue and demonstrated a standout among the most investigated innovations by human services offices on account of its essential job and wide scope of utilization in clinical sciences. WBAN includes correspondence between little sensor hubs with every now and again evolving condition, consequently a bunch of issues will be taken care of. A portion of the serious issues are physical layer issues, interoperability and versatility issues, dependability, asset the executives, ease of use, energy utilization, and QoS (quality of service) issues. This exploration chapter incorporates an extensive overview of late patterns in WBAN and gives forthcoming answers for some serious issues utilizing intellectual methodology and a proposed idea of cognitive radio–based WBAN engineering. Hence, a traditional WBAN engineering can be ad-libbed to a versatile, increasingly dependable, and proficient WBAN framework utilizing cognition-based methodology.

WBAN is a remote system's administration innovation, in view of radio frequency (RF) that interconnects various little hubs with sensor or actuator capacities. These hubs work in close contact to, on or couple of centimeters inside, a human body, to help different restorative region and nonmedicinal territory applications.[1] WBAN innovation is profoundly refreshing in the field of medicinal science and human social insurance.[2-5] Additionally, huge commitment is conveyed in the field of biomedical and other logical regions.[6] Also, its applications are broad in nonrestorative territories such as consumer gadgets and individual diversion.

A great deal of research work is being done on WBANs. The primary issues concentrated upon are size of system, result precision, hub thickness, control supply, versatility, information rate, vitality utilization, QoS, and real-time correspondence. WBAN hubs use scaled down batteries because of their little size. Thus, the system must work and perform in a power productive way with the goal that the existence term of intensity sources can be augmented. A large portion of the work in this specific space has been on advancement of better MAC (media access control address) conventions for vitality effective preparing. By and by, there are two distinct methodologies of MAC convention planning for sensor systems. Initial one is contention-based MAC convention plan. This sort of MAC convention is called carrier sense multiple access—collision avoidance (CSMA/CA). This structure has its hubs needs for channel access before transmitting information. The advantages of CSMA/CA-based conventions incorporate no time synchronization limitations, simple flexibility to arrange varieties and versatility. The other methodology is schedule-based MAC convention. Case of this sort of convention is TDMA (time-division multiple access) based, in which time-opened access to the channel is given. Henceforth, various clients get isolated availabilities for information transmission. These openings can be of fixed or variable length. Schedule vacancy controller is utilized for giving availabilities.

The advantages of this methodology are diminished inactive tuning in, overheading, and impact. TDMA-based methodology is utilized in vitality effective MAC convention.[21] A tale approach of heartbeat fueled the MAC convention is given by Ref. [27]. This convention is TDMA based and utilized for body sensor systems. The work incorporates use of heartbeat mood to perform time synchronization and consequently gives a vitality proficient MAC layer by evading power utilization related with time synchronization reference point transmission. Utilizing a robot to revive batteries and exchange information can drastically build the life expectancy of a remote sensor arrange. In this, the way of the robot is constrained by waypoints, and the districts where every sensor can be adjusted are featured. We utilize a blend of angle drop and a "numerous voyaging sales rep issue" look calculation to move the waypoints toward districts where sensor hubs can be revived while guaranteeing waypoints remain near one another.

An auxiliary well-being remote sensor arrange (Wireless Sensor Network (WSN)) should keep going for quite a long time, yet conventional dispensable batteries cannot continue such a system. Vitality is the significant obstruction to supportability of WSNs. Most vitality is devoured by (1) remote transmissions of saw information and (2) long-removed multijump transmissions from the source sensors to the sink. This chapter investigates how to misuse developing remote power exchange innovation by utilizing automated unmanned vehicles (UVs) to support the WSNs. These UVs slice information transmissions from long to short separations, gather detected data, and recharge WSN's vitality.

2.2 APPLICATIONS TO HEALTHCARE

2.2.1 HEALTH MONITORING SYSTEM

Internet of Things (IoT) has increased tremendous fame in medical because of its capacity to have applications for which the administrations can be conveyed to shoppers quickly at insignificant expense. An imperative application is the utilization of IoT and cloud innovations to help specialists in giving increasingly successful demonstrative procedures.

Specifically, here we examine electrocardiogram (ECG) information investigation utilizing IoT and the cloud. The slender improvement of Internet availability and its openness to any gadget has made IoT an appealing alternative for creating well being–observing frameworks.

ECG information examination and observing comprise a situation that normally appropriates into such situation. ECG represents the important appearance of the contractile action of myocardium of the heart. Such action conveys an exact wave that is reiterated after some phase and that addresses the heart rate. The examination of the condition of the ECG signal is accustomed to perceive problems and is the most broadly perceived procedure to deal with distinguish coronary ailment. IoT advancements permit the remote checking of a patient's heart rate, examination in real time, and notice the therapeutic guide workforce and experts should these data reveal possibly unsafe situations.[1] Thus, a patient in threat can be checked without embarking to an emergency center for ECG examination. Meanwhile, experts and emergency treatment can immediately be informed with respect to cases that require their assistance.

From Figure 2.1, we conclude that a champion among the most characteristic points of interest of disseminated registering for human administrations is that the environment cloud makes it distant less complex to account and usage of getting information and helpful pictures.[8] The better method to manage the information will progress get to, proliferation accumulating limit, and lift safety. Various specialists find disseminated figuring creates it suitable to cooperate and deal thought as a gathering. Over and done with phones and submissions manufactured unequivocally for social protection affiliations, the IoT speeds things up and provides better correspondence at a distance.

Nation care and calamity reaction become progressively down to earth. Huge data have transformed into a marvelous test for some prosperity affiliations, and the cloud empowers providers to set aside some money by constraining in-house accumulating needs. The information in such as manner ends up being progressively open from various zones, and paying little heed to in the case of something happens close by, the data are up till now defended. A champion among the most charming fields of disseminated processing is data examination.[2] By following and handling information in the IoT, logically, suppliers can "procure" it for therapeutic exploration, transfer age, design noticing, and progressively modified thought.

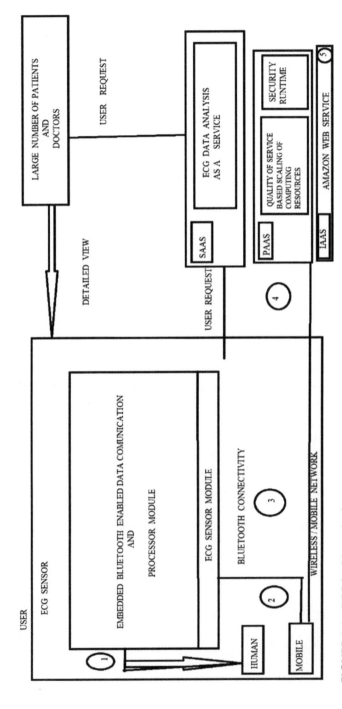

FIGURE 2.1 ECG health monitoring system.

Human administrations affiliations can join these advancements and adequately distribute data to make much continuously thorough gigantic data pools for to pick up from in greater, progressively multifaceted systems.³³ The cloud enables a lot of ground-breaking data answers for superpower the investigation technique. Tremendous data used to be awfully sweeping for humbler PCs to manage, yet through the moved figuring force of the cloud, using these goliath educational accumulations for progression transforms into a reality. It thusly winds up more straightforward and even more expensive to improve various types prescriptions, and it specially indicates stimulating potential results concerning DNA ordering.

2.2.2 REMOTE STEADY ECG CHECKING

Holter watching is a basic fragment of the telemedicine. Nowadays, there are a few techniques for the ECG Holter trading the information to the center as follow:

Connect the ECG banner to the area PC truly, by then the banner will get examined through the master therapeutic staff from emergency facility. This represents a strategy of instrument in restorative facility. With everything taken into account, the instrument is simply in the center since many patients cannot deal with the expense of the equipment.³ Save the ECG banner to the area memory storing. The patients or their relatives take the memory storing to the restorative facility to be dissected by an expert. Such philosophy is employed for the flexible ECG monitor, yet the data may set aside such a long exertion to be sent to the emergency facility that the patients may miss the best time for treatment. Through the Web, it trades the ECG data to the remote checking center. Thusly, you ought to have the Web, so this philosophy obliged the degree of use.⁸

2.2.3 TELEMEDICINE INNOVATION

By virtue of the cloud, high-tech devices, and convenient advancement, giving social protection from a partition has transformed into a reality. Models consolidate discourses, teletherapeutic techniques, and checking patients without having them come in. Still dubious absolutely how to utilize the cloud for better execution? Need to get acquainted with the upsides of conveyed processing for social protection? Interact with one of our authorities to discuss what is possible or get some answers concerning other tech game plans that look good for affiliations such as yours.[7] The area by then analyzes the executed structure and how it capacities with the help of test framework and hardware stages. It wires answers for a couple of issues related with IoT and shows how they work in the realized structure for its particular stages. The results show that the structure limits effectively on both test framework condition and hardware systems and can be executed in a facility environment.

The Web of things (WoT) advancement is wrapping up dynamically normal in the human administrations industry. The fundamental usages of IoT in the area of smart medication consolidate the view of the organization, digitization of restorative data, and of the remedial methodology. Telemedicine watching generally uses progresses related to the WoT development to collect a patient-driven, remote gathering, and constant checking organization structure focused on helping essentially missed out patients.[8] The main inspiration driving arranging telemedicine watching advancement was to diminish the amount of patients entering restorative facilities and focuses.

As per the Centers for Disease Control and Prevention, around 50% of Americans possess atleast one incessant ailment, and their treatment expenditures represent more than 75% of the country's USD 2 trillion in restorative uses. Notwithstanding the mind-boggling expense of cutting edge treatment and medical procedure, specialists spend approximately billions of dollars on routine checks, research facility tests, and other observing administrations. With the progression of telemedicine innovation, refined sensors get utilized to screen patients with constant updates.

Moreover, the focal point of telemedicine observing has step-by-step moved from improving ways of life to rapidly giving lifesaving data and to medicinal projects concentrated on instructive trade. In viable applications, well-being data of patients can be transmitted through the Web, improving the nature of restorative administrations. This innovation likewise enables specialists to direct virtual counsels and give scholarly help to different medical clinics by specialists from a substantial emergency clinic. This will stretch out astounding restorative assets to essential human services foundations, help build up a long haul, ceaseless instruction administration framework for clinical cases, and improve the nature of proceeding with training for essential social insurance laborers.

Application of the Internet of Things (IoT)   39

Utilizing the RFID (radio frequency identification) innovation, the specialist can take the bedside test effectively. They can recognize the person's ID; if there are a few blunders, the alarm will call the specialist automatically. The RFID innovation connected in blood the executives can viably keep away from the inadequacies of little limit scanner tags, accomplish noncontact distinguishing proof, decrease blood pollution, and improve information accumulation proficiency.[8] Beside the RFID, there are numerous sensors in the patient's room that can catch the data of the patients and exchange the information to the specialist in the medical clinic. In this connection, Figure 2.2 illustrates a scenario of smart service.

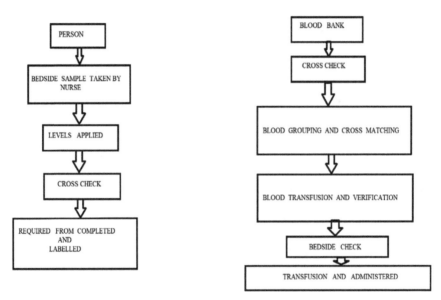

FIGURE 2.2   Smart service.

2.2.4   RFID APPLICATIONS TO ASSIST THE ELDERLY LIVE INDEPENDENTLY

PC researchers at the University of Adelaide are driving an undertaking to grow new RFID sensor frameworks, which helps more seasoned individuals with the goal that they can securely remain autonomous. Scientists utilized RFID and sensor innovation to distinguish and screen individuals' exercises consequently. This can assist with both routine consideration and emergency care on account of a mishap inside the home. Also, the framework includes low information costs and no necessities for escalated testing. Despite a maturing populace, this application has huge potential. Holter observing is a critical part of the medicine industry.[7]

The patients take the memory stockpiling to the emergency clinic to be analyzed by a specialist. This methodology is utilized for the compact ECG monitor, yet the information may set aside such an extended effort to be sent to the emergency clinic which the patients may miss the best time for treatment. Through the web exchange, the ECG information to the remote checking is focused on. Along these lines, you should have the Web, so this methodology constrained the extent of use. Through remote systems, exchange of the information to the observing focus is done.[9]

Mobile correspondences innovation from the recent 2.5-age CDMA and GPRS to the third era portable interchanges improvement, with the 3G correspondence innovation and advance the utilization of progressively complex, 3G versatile correspondence innovation in cardiovascular. Remote zones of social insurance assume a gigantic job.[6]

2.2.5 SMART WHEELCHAIR USES

The assignment of shrewd wheelchair innovation is to securely and serenely convey the client to a goal. Amid use, the wheelchair requires acknowledging the client's guidance, yet it additionally needs to begin its obstruction shirking, route, and other practical modules because of natural data. Dissimilar to a self-propelled versatile robot, the wheelchair and the client are a cooperative framework. Various factors, for example, plan, security, solace, and simplicity of activity, are (or if nothing else ought to be) the most basic factors in savvy wheelchair design. Differences in potential clients' physical abilities imply that smart wheelchair configuration should likewise be adaptable and secluded. Every client ought to have the capacity to pick the right modules by their sort and level of inability.

Utilitarian modules ought to be both removable as well as replaceable, with the goal that wheelchair work is modifiable as well-being levels change. The general capacity of the savvy wheelchair gets isolated into the accompanying subcapacities: natural observation and route capacities, control capacities, driving capacities, and human–PC communication.

Through the utilitarian investigation and modularization of the smart wheelchair's highlights combined with explicit research outcomes, the framework will probably comprise of three principle parts: the sensor module, the drive control module, and the human interface module.

The sensor module would comprise of two sections—interior state discernment and outer condition observation. The frame of mind sensor decides the mentality and location data of the wheelchair. The removal speed and separation of the encoder gives oneself situating data. Visual, ultrasonic, and closeness switches are essentially in charge of ceaselessly getting data about impediments. For the drive control module, back wheel arrangement of an engine would be utilized with standard electric wheelchair control tasks—front, back, left, and right. Human–PC cooperation is either finished with physical controls, for example, a joystick or mouth stick or keyboard controls, for example, a PC. A savvy wheelchair has two autonomous drive wheels, each outfitted with an engine controller. The constant location information of the two engine controllers structures the odometer, relatively situating the sensor. The establishment of the tendency sensor and the whirligig is carried out to quantify the stance condition of the wheelchair amid the voyaging procedure.

Ultrasonic sensors and vicinity switches acquire encompassing data. For accomplishing a more extensive scope of snag data, eight infrared sensors and eight ultrasonic sensors are outfitted with the framework. Likewise, establishment of a CCD (charge-coupled device) camera is carried out to decide profundity data before the seat. Moreover, the savvy wheelchair can adjust exclusively on two wheels. This unmistakable element necessitates that the wheelchair gets worked with a remarkable structure dependent on driving each wheel by a different DC engine and keeping the equalization of the seat's weight straightforwardly over the wheels on a solitary hub. This is accomplished by using sensors to decide the pitch and yaw, accordingly, deciding the demeanor of the seat progressively. Signs from the sensors move to the seat's processor that runs the data by a control calculation to decide the ideal speed and bearing for each wheel to keep up parity while pushing ahead or in reverse.

The savvy wheelchair utilizes a blend of a tilt sensor and a spinner to shape a disposition sensor fit for deciding the wheelchair's frame of mind as it traversed a plane. The utilization of the tilt sensor is to decide the wheelchair's level of deviation from vertical, while the spinner decides its precise speed.

We have to prepare a circuit configuration in low cost and in efficient manner. Figure 2.3 represent a scenario of circuit configuration. If the device is of high cost, then middle-class people cannot buy or use it.

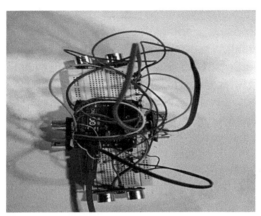

FIGURE 2.3 Circuit configuration.

2.2.6 PORTABLE MEDICINE

By estimating indispensable signs, for example, body temperature and pulse, and shaping an individual restorative plan for every patient including weight, level of cholesterol in the body, muscle-to-fat ratio, and protein ratio, we can dissect the patient's general physical and mental situation and return physiological marker information to the patient's locale, guardian, or related medicinal association.[11] It enables the patient to create convenient amendments to concerned eating regimen, encourages the age of specialized customized therapeutic exhortation, and gives examine information to emergency clinics and research foundations.

2.2.7 UTILIZATIONS OF RFID WRISTBANDS

Soon every individual's phone will resemble a private specialist. While everybody absolutely has their own involvement with these issues, it is normal in China to see large queues of patients—hanging tight to take an enlistment number and see a specialist. Patients can be overpowered by visits, as emergency clinics are overflowed with thousands or a huge number of outpatients in a typical day. All in all, how does this framework work? At the point when an individual turns out to be sick, the person in question needs to see a specialist. Thus, by what means can we proficiently support everybody? This should be possible correctly by empowering these sorts of changes as we enter what is to come.[10]

Experience makes a specialist, and this experience is aggregated by watching information pointers identified with the patient's sickness. In the event that a specialist's experience can be accumulated into a database, at that point, the patient should simply to enter his or her information markers into the framework.[12] At the point when the parameters in the database have achieved an adequate dimension, the database will almost certainly play out a programmed conclusion. At last, the database turns into a sort of "robot master." These databases work by gathering a sufficient measure of the master's disease cases, consolidating them to frame information pointers and, in this way, producing a database demonstrate.

For instance, on the off chance that we have the information markers for the cure of 10,000 instances of leukemia, at that point, the database holds 10,000 answers for treating leukemia. This sort of database will in the long run change into an inherent programming in our PDAs, expanding the portability of medications.[13] In the event that the product is unfit to evaluate the circumstance proficiently, at that point a human master will almost certainly regulate treatment over the Web. In time, every one of us will have his or her own "private robot specialist" living on concerned telephone numbers.

2.2.8 GPS POSITIONING APPLICATIONS FOR PATIENTS WITH HEART DISEASE

Every individual requires to construct their well-being database. On the off chance that a sufferer of coronary illness has made their advanced well-being record, at that point, when their heart starts to act strangely or represents an impending danger, the applicable information will be promptly passed to the framework that can utilize GPS situating to call the vital emergency administrations from the closest medical clinic.[14] This might be a basic IoT application, and at the same time, later on, we may all have our own registration gadgets at home.

We should simply put our palm on the gadget that will at that point gather circulatory strain, pulse, heartbeat, and body temperature. Later on, it may even have the capacity to perform compound tests.[15] This information will be consequently passed to the emergency clinic's server farm, and, if fundamental, a specialist will request that we come into the medical clinic for further assessment or go to a nearby health center to get treatment.

2.2.9 WELL-BEING ID CARD

When we take the metro, pretty much everything can get practiced with the swipe of a card. This makes the whole experience substantially more helpful for most of clients. In therapeutic IoT field, seeing a specialist ought to be like taking the metro. Throughout medicinal treatment, the client's authentic ID card is the main legitimate verification of character and should get filtered on a card scanner, with the patient presenting a specific measure of cash as an initial instalment.[16] In no time flat, the computerized card scanner/author would then be able to deliver a "RFID Visit Card" (this could likewise serve as a protection card) that the patient can use to get an enlistment number for seeing the specialist. When the patient has a card, they can go to see a specialist at any treatment focus.

At the treatment focus, the framework will consequently enter their data into the comparing specialist's workstation. All through treatment, data identified with the specialist issuing examinations, medication, and other treatment data gets passed on to the proper divisions.[17] For whatever length of time that the patient has their "RFID Visit Card," the card scanner/author at the relating office can check the majority of this data, issue prescription, and manage treatment without requiring the patient to keep running back and forth figuring and paying installments. When the method is finished, the expense printer prints out a receipt and cost list.

Additionally, identified with "RFID Visit Cards," medical clinics will almost certainly give in patients a "RFID wristband" that will incorporate the patient's name, sexual orientation, age, calling, registration time, conclusion time, examination time, and charge data. The achievement of acquiring the patient's personal data completes with no manual error, and the encryption of patient's profiles is expected to ensure their security. This guarantees the wristband as the main wellspring of the patient's recognizable proof data and keeps away from human blunder due to manual error. Besides, these wristbands will likewise incorporate location tracking, making it impossible for the wearer to escape the emergency clinic.

On the off chance that a patient coercively removes their "RFID wristband" or leaves a specific range around the medical clinic, at that point, the framework will issue an alarm, setting off an assessment of the wearer's crucial signs (breathing, pulse, beat) and decide the patient's "danger level" in light of that data. The framework will probably assess physiological changes 24 h/day, and, when the wearer's danger level achieves a specific edge, an alarm will be issued consequently to permit medical clinic staff to react as quickly as time permits.

Examination, imaging, medical procedure, sedate organization, and different assignments normal to the treatment procedure are altogether encouraged by affirming persistent data through their "RFID wristband" and recording the time that each progression in the process starts. This guarantees medical attendants and emergency clinic examination staff at each dimension in controlling the proper consideration without mistake, in this way, giving the nature of the whole treatment process. The patient can utilize their "RFID wristband" to check their treatment expenses and explicit card perusing machines. They can likewise print their charge results, protection plans, tenets and guidelines, nursing directions, treatment plan, and medication data. This will serve to expand the patient's capacity to effectively get their treatment data and increment generally speaking patient fulfilment.[18]

2.2.10 THERAPEUTIC TOOLS AND MEDICINE OBSERVING AND SMART ADMINISTRATION

Due to the advancement of RFIDs, IoT have begun to catch increasingly broad solicitations in the field of restorative organization portrayal. Advancement of IoT can help avoid general medicinal issues by helping in the generation, conveyance, and following of therapeutic instruments and prescription. This assembles the idea of medicinal management while diminishing organization prices.

As per the World Wellbeing Association, the proportion of phony prescriptions on the planet indicates more than 12% of offers of the medicines the world over. Accordingly, RFID innovation will assume a fundamental job in the following and checking of medications and hardware and the guideline of the market for medicinal goods. In particular, IoT innovation in the area of administration has presentations in the accompanying zones.[19]

2.2.11 PHARMACEUTICAL COUNTERFEIT DEVICE PREDICTION

It appended to an item will have an interesting idea that is very hard to fashion. This will assume a fundamental job in confirmation of data and hostile to falsifying, demonstrating a successful measurement against restorative misrepresentation. For instance, it will be conceivable to spread tranquilize data to an open database from which an emergency clinic can verify the substance of the mark in contradiction of the data in the database to effortlessly distinguish possible fakes.

2.2.12 REAL-TIME OBSERVING

The whole generation procedure can use RFID labels to achieve thorough item observing. This is particularly vital when the item gets sent. A scan introduced on the generation line can automatically recognize each medication's data and spread it to the databank as the item becomes bundled. Amid the conveyance procedure, any middle of the road data gets recorded whenever implying that it is conceivable to screen from start to finish.

2.2.13 RESTORATIVE WASTE MANAGEMENT INFORMATION

Collaboration by emergency clinics and delivery organizations will help to set up a discernible therapeutic unused following framework utilizing RFID innovation. This will guarantee that the therapeutic unused gets appropriately ecstatic to the dealing plant and will keep the unlawful dumping of bio hazardous medicinal waste.

2.3 IoT AND ADVANCED MEDICAL MANAGEMENT

IoT has wide presentation predictions in the area of therapeutic data they executive. At present, the interest for medicinal data and the executives in emergency clinics are essentially in the accompanying angles: ID, test acknowledgment, and restorative record recognizable proof. Recognizable proof incorporates patient ID, doctor ID, test ID (counting drug distinguishing proof), medicinal hardware ID, research facility ID, and restorative record ID (counting side effects and ID of ailment).[20]

Application of the Internet of Things (IoT)   47

We can separate explicit applications into the following accompanying territories:

2.3.1   PERSISTENT STATISTICS MANAGEMENT

The patient's family restorative past data, the patient's medicinal history, different inspections, therapeutic data, medicate hypersensitivities, and other well-being documents can help specialists to create disease handling programs. Specialists and medical attendants can quantify the patient's essential signatures, and, amid medicines, for example, chemotherapy, they can utilize ongoing observing data to wipe out the utilization of wrong medications and that can automatically remind medical caretakers to do sedate verification and other works.

2.3.2   SMART MEDICINAL MANAGEMENT

There are some unordinary conditions, for example, when there are vast quantities of setbacks, a failure to achieve relatives, or the basically sick. In such situations, RFID advancements' solid and proficient stockpiling and testing techniques will help with the quick recognizable proof of pertinent subtleties, for example, the patient's biodata like name, age, blood classification, and past restorative past information. This will accelerate confirmation systems for emergency patients and leave all the more valuable period for management. Of specific significance are the establishments of 4G video hardware in ambulances. As affected people are headed to the medical clinic, the emergency room is now receiving acquainted with the patient's condition and can viably plan for emergency salvation. In the event that the area is a long way from the clinic, there is a likelihood of utilizing medicinal imaging frameworks as a major aspect of the emergency salvation method.

2.3.3   MEDICATION STORAGE MANAGEMENT

RFID innovation can mechanize the entire hawser of capacity and investigation to decrease the obligatory operational hours that recently got laid on broadsheet. It also avoids store deficiencies and encourages the review of medications. It can likewise support to keep away from perplexity emerging from comparable medication names or dose sum and measurement type. In general, it will reinforce sedate administration and guarantee that prescriptions get gave and arranged immediately.

2.3.4   QUIET INFORMATION MANAGEMENT

Smart use of RFID innovation to donation of blood center administration can successfully maintain a strategic distance from the inconveniences of scanner tags having restricted data limit and can understand the objective of contactless distinguishing proof, lessen blood defilement, acknowledge multitarget recognizable proof, and improve information gathering productivity.

2.3.5   BATTLING PHARMACEUTICAL ERROR

Data board in the drug store will guarantee that prescription is effectively conveyed and gotten. To date, drug store as of now gets actualized in such angles as giving solutions, changing measurements, nursing organization, quiet utilization of prescription, viability following, stock administration, buy of provisions, conservation of natural conditions, and assurance of time span of usability. It is likewise cast off to affirm which sort of medication is endorsed to the sick person, and not just the data of which tranquilizer the patient is taking and whether they have taken in it yet and even which part number the medication originated from. This keeps away from the likelihood of patients missing doses and, in case of a superiority control issue, influenced patients getting recognized rapidly.

2.3.6   MEDICINAL INSTRUMENT AND DRUG MONITORING AND MANAGEMENT

2.3.6.1   RESTORATIVE DEVICE AND PHARMACEUTICALS ANTICOUNTERFEITING

The name appended to an item will have an exceptional character that is very hard to produce. This will assume a basic job in checking of data and resist falsification, demonstrating a viable duplicate product-measurement against medicinal extortion. Sometimes, it must be conceivable to diffuse sedate data to an open data storehouse from which a patient or emergency clinic can verify the substance of the mark in contradiction of the information in the database to effortlessly recognize prospective fakes.

2.3.6.2 THERAPEUTIC WASTE INFORMATION MANAGEMENT

Participation by emergency clinics and conveyance of organizations will support set up a detectable therapeutic surplus following framework utilizing RFID innovation. This will guarantee that the medicinal waste gets legitimately conveyance to the treatment plant and will keep the unlawful discarding of bio unsafe therapeutic waste.

2.3.7 ADVANCED SMART MEDICAL

WoT has wide request prospects in the area of medicinal data board. At present, the interest for therapeutic data board in clinics is mostly in the accompanying perspectives: distinguishing proof, example acknowledgment, and restorative record ID. Recognizable proof incorporates quiet distinguishing proof, doctor ID, test ID (counting drug ID), medicinal gear ID, research facility ID, and restorative record ID (counting manifestations and ID of illness).

2.4 EPLICIT APPLICATIONS OF IOT IN SMART HEALTHCARE

We can partition explicit applications into the following accompanying regions:

2.4.1 PATIENT DATA MANAGEMENT

The patient's family medicinal data, the patient's therapeutic past, different inspections, restorative data, medicate sensitivities, and various electronic well-being documents can help specialists to create management programs.[21] Specialists and medical caretakers can quantify the patient's fundamental symbol, and, amid medications, for example, chemotherapy, they can utilize continuous observing data to kill the utilization of incorrect drugs or off beam needles that can automatically repeat attendants to complete medication patterned and various work.

2.4.2 MEDICINAL BACKUP ADMINISTRATION

There are some uncommon conditions, for example, when there are vast quantities of losses, a powerlessness to achieve relatives, or the fundamentally patient. In such situations, RFID advancements' solid and proficient stockpiling and testing strategies will help with the fast distinguishing proof of important subtleties, for example, the patient's data (i.e., name, age, blood classification) emergency information, and past restorative past data. This will accelerate confirmation methods for emergency patients and leave all the more valuable time for management.[22]

As patients are en route to the clinic, the emergency room is as of now receiving acquainted with the condition of sick people and can successfully get ready for emergency salvation. On the off chance that the area is a long way from the clinic, there is a likelihood of utilizing therapeutic frameworks as a major aspect of the emergency salvation process. Innovation of RFID can computerize the entire cable of capacity and assessment to lessen the vital working periods and rationalize forms that recently got led on broadsheet. It can help forestall run of the mill deficiencies and encourage the review of medications. It can likewise help to maintain a strategic distance from perplexity emerging from comparable medication names or measurement sum and dose type. In general, it will reinforce and tranquilize the executives and guarantee that medications are given and arranged immediately.[23]

2.4.3 QUIET EVIDENCE CONTROLLING

The use of RFID innovation to blood donation center administration may viably maintain a strategic distance from the disservices of scanner tags having constrained data limit and can understand the objective of contactless ID, decrease blood tainting, acknowledge multitarget recognizable proof, and improve information accumulation productivity.

2.4.4 BATTLING PHARMACEUTICAL ERROR

Data executives in the drug store will guarantee that medication is effectively disseminated and gotten. To date, drug store data is as board as of now it gets actualized in such viewpoints as giving solutions, altering doses, nursing organization, understanding utilization of medicine, viability following, stock administration, buy of provisions, conservation of ecological conditions, and assurance of timeframe of realistic usability and additionally, used to affirm which kind of medication gets endorsed to the patient, and to not just top score which tranquilize the patients are captivating and whether they have occupied in it however, even which part amount the medication originated from.[24] This keeps away from the likelihood of patients missing planned drugs, and, in case of a quality control issue, influenced long-sufferings get recognized rapidly.

2.4.5 MEDICINAL APPARATUS AND DRUG TRACKING

By precisely, sound tracking things and longsuffering characters and giving solid help to mishap taking care of, accessible restorative gadgets and drug are represented. By precisely recording fundamental data, for example, item use, unfavorable occasions, regions where excellence control issues may happen, patients getting included and areas of idle items, anyone can trace and deal with wrong items.

2.4.6 ASSOCIATED INFORMATION SHARING

To start with, structure a very much created and incorporated medicinal system through the sharing of restorative data and records.[25] From one viewpoint, approved specialists can check the medicinal history of the patient, past experience of ailment, action, and protection subtleties. Patients will likewise have the opportunity to pick or supplant specialists and medical clinics. Then again, community and provincial medical clinics can consistently interface with focal emergency clinics for data and specialized master guidance, just as organizing referrals and get preparing.

2.4.7 PREDICTION OF PROTEIN STRUCTURE

Solicitations in science frequently necessitate high registering abilities and regularly work on huge informational indexes that reason broad I/O activities. Due to these necessities, science applications have regularly utilized supercomputing and bunch registering frameworks. Comparable capabilities can be utilized on interest utilizing distributed calculating advances in a progressively unique manner, therefore opening new open doors for bioinformatics applications. Structure of protein forecast is a serious errand that is principal to various kinds of investigation in the existing knowledges.

The arrangement of a protein cannot be straightforwardly induced from the grouping of qualities that form its construction; however, it is the aftereffect of compound calculations went for recognizing the arrangement that limits the necessitated vitality. This errand necessitates examination of a space with an enormous number of states, subsequently making an extensive number of calculations for every one of these phases.

The computational influence needed for construction of protein expectation would now be able to be obtained on interest, without owning a bunch or exploring the organization to gain admittance to parallel and conveyed figuring facilities.[33] Cloud processing presents access to such limit on a compensation for each utilization premise. One system that examines the utilization of cloud innovations for protein structure forecast is Jeeva—a coordinated web entryway that empowers researchers to offload the expectation errand to a processing cloud based on Aneka platform. The expectation task utilizes AI techniques (support vector machines) for deciding these optional structures of proteins.

These systems make an interpretation of the issue into one of example recognition, whereas arrangement must be characterized into one of three conceivable parts (E, H, and C). A famous usage dependent on help of vector machines separates the example acknowledgment issue into three phases: instatement, order, and a last stage. Despite the fact that these three stages must be computed in sequence, it is conceivable to exploit equivalent execution in the characterization stage, where various classifiers are executed parallel. This makes the chance to reasonably lessen the computational time of the assumption. The expectation algorithms then converted into an errand chart that is succumbed to Aneka.[26]

Application of the Internet of Things (IoT)

When this type of assignment is completed, the center product makes there results accessible for perception done through the entryway. The upside of utilizing cloud technologies versus customary matrix frameworks is the capacity to use an adaptable registering foundation that can be developed and contracted on demand. This idea is particular of cloud advances and establishes a key favorable position when tenders are obtainable and conveyed as an administration. By analyzing Jeeva Portal, we can find it carefully predict final structure, initial phase, classification phase, final phase, task graph, and Aneka. The notation used in Figure 2.4 is depicted here.

- A: BLAST
- B: CONSTRUCT DATA VECTOR
- C: HH CLASSIFIER
- D: SS CLASSIFIER
- E: TT CLASSIFIER
- F: HS CLASSIFIER
- G: ST CLASSIFIER
- H: TH CLASSIFIER
- I: PREDICT FINAL SECONDARY STRUCTURE

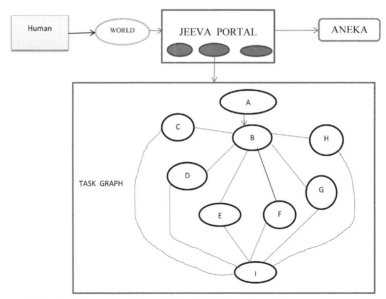

FIGURE 2.4 Architecture and description of the Jeeva Portal.

Figure 2.5 describes the scalable nature of classifier, and the dynamic platform, that is, Aneka, provides a distinctive offer. Quality enunciation describing is the estimation of articulation measurements of qualities without a moment's delay. It is used to grasp the regular methodology that is initiated by therapeutic treatment at a cell level. Protein structure prediction activity is a key piece of medicine plan, since it empowers scientists to recognize the effects of a specific treatment. Another basic utilization of value enunciation profiling is malady assurance and treatment. Harmful development is an ailment depicted by uncontrolled cell advancement and proliferation. This thing directly occurs in light of the way that characteristics controlling the telephone improvement mutate.

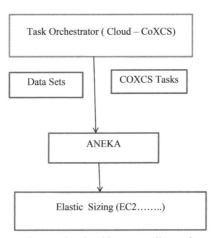

FIGURE 2.5 Data processing on the cloud in cancer diagnosis.

This infers that all the cancer-causing cells contain changed genes. In this context, gene verbalization profiling is utilized to give a logically accurate request of tumors. The game plan of value explanation data tests into specific classes is a challenging task. The dimensionality of ordinary quality enunciation datasets ranges from a couple of thousands to more than incalculable characteristics. However, simply little precedent sizes are routinely open for examination. This issue is as often as possible moved nearer with learning classifiers, which quality rate of masses of condition-action choice that controls the course of action system. The extended classifier system is adequately utilized for masterminding huge datasets in the bioinformatics and programming designing spaces.

Application of the Internet of Things (IoT) 55

However, the reasonability of XCS, when went facing with high-dimensional data (such as quality enunciation datasets), has not been explored in point. An assortment of this computation, CoXCS,[27] has ended up being effective in these conditions. CoXCS parcels the entire interest space into subdomains and uses the standard XCS estimation in each of these subdomains. Such a system is computationally raised anyway and can be successfully parallelized in light of the way that the portrayals issues on the subdomains can be handled simultaneously. Cloud-CoXCS is a cloud-based use of CoXCS that impacts the platform called Aneka to deal with the gathering issues in equivalent and make their conclusions.

The count is compelled by procedures, which describe the way wherein the outcomes are collected and whether the strategy ought to be repeated in infant antikidnapping system. At an extensive general medical clinic's obstetrics and gynecology office or a ladies and youngsters' emergency clinic, joining mother and tyke distinguishing proof administration, and newborn child security, the executives will avert unsupervised access by pariahs. Specifically, every infant ought to get a RFID anklet that remarkably distinguishes child and has a novel correspondence with own parent's data. To decide whether the personnel has the right infant, the smart anklet (using RFID) just needs to get investigated by an attendant.

2.4.8 ALERT AREA

From constant checking and following clinic medicinal gadgets, the framework will automatically invite for support in case of patient pain. It will likewise keep patients from visiting the medical clinic all alone and will keep the harm or burglary of costly gadgets and secure temperature-delicate medications and research facility tests.[28]

2.5 SPECIALIZED PROBLEMS FACING MEDICAL IOT

In this medicinal area, irrespective to anything, we have to report numerous specialized issues confronting IoT.

2.5.1 NODE VERSATILITY AND DYNAMIC LARGE SCALE SYSTEM: THE BOARD IN ENORMOUS SCALE SYSTEMS

At the point where there is a development of the observing framework to protect private networks, urban groups, or whole nations, the span of the system will overpower, and checking hubs will all must be portable somewhat. Along these lines, we need to plan a proper system topology, the executive's structure, and system portability for the board strategies.[29]

2.5.2 INFORMATION COMPLETENESS AND DATA COMPRESSION

Hubs will now and again need to direct observation for 24 h every day, gathering a huge measure of data that should be put away utilizing a pressure calculation to decrease stockpiling and transmission volume. In any case, conventional information pressure calculations are unreasonably exorbitant for sensor hubs. Moreover, pressure calculations cannot lose the first information. Additionally, the framework could misdiagnose the patient's condition. We use many data centers, producing large amount of carbon. So it is very important to reduce power and carbon emission for a green environment.[30]

From Figure 2.6, we presume that server farms are costly to keep up, yet additionally hostile to nature. Carbon discharge because of server farm is an overall issue. High vitality costs and gigantic carbon emissions are caused because of the monstrous measure of power expected to power and cool the various servers facilitated in this information center. Cloud specialist co-ops need to embrace measures to guarantee that their overall revenue is not significantly diminished because of high vitality costs.[31]

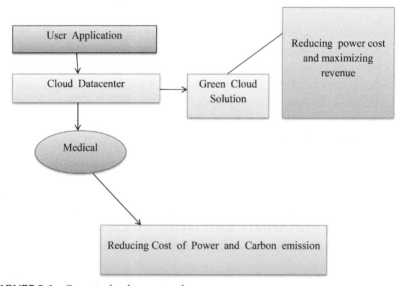

FIGURE 2.6 Green technology scenario.

Figure 2.7 shows that bringing down the vitality utilization of server farms is a difficult and complex issue as figuring applications and the information are developing so faster that bigger servers and plates are anticipated to process them quick enough inside the desired timeframe. IoT is imagined to carry out not just proficient preparing and use of figuring framework, yet in addition to limit vitality utilization. This is fundamental for guaranteeing that the further enhancement of IoT is reasonable. IoT, with progressively unavoidable front-end customer gadgets, for example, iPhones associating with back-end information centers will cause a colossal heightening of vitality utilization. To address this issue, server farm assets should be overseen in a vitality productive way to drive green IoT.[32] In particular, cloud assets should be apportioned not exclusively to fulfill QoS prerequisites determined by clients by means of administration level agreements, yet in addition to lessening vitality usage. This can get accomplished by putting market-based utility models to acknowledge client demands, which can be of satisfaction to improve income alongside vitality, which is an effective use of IoT foundation.

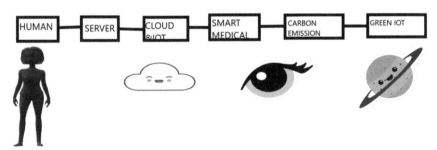

FIGURE 2.7 Protocol of green environment scenario.

2.5.3 INFORMATION SECURITY

Remote sensors arrange hubs structure, a self-composed system which is defenseless against assaults and are, clearly, dangerous when managing patient data that must be kept private. The processing intensity of a sensor hub is very lacking. Subsequently, conventional protection and hiding innovations are not appropriate to this type of situations. The use of IoT is expanding step by step in each part of the medicinal services industry. In this article, we have investigated different utilizations of IoT in the therapeutic business.

2.5.4 DUPLICATE MEDICINE DETECTION

Duplicate medicine is very hazardous to our health. It is an unquestionable actuality that fake items provide risks to the organizations worldwide over disregarding patent rights and causing tremendous business losses. Thus, it is essential for firms beyond any doubt that they curb duplication. Existing innovations for electrical manufactured find include for applying of additional security looks incline toward Watermark Technology to the token stock itself that raises the charges of one's product. In this chapter, a solid technique for fake expectation is proposed. This strategy can be utilized by client to foresee fake for their everyday need things accessible in the market. Presently the development of new versions of the item dependably accompanies the danger of faking, now and again that could influence the organization's goodwill.

We have utilized the idea of undetectable and unmistakable watermarking present in thing itself to give credibility of the product. This is an ease arrangement that enables endeavors and buyers to recognize the legitimacy of item. Because of the quick data terminating in present day time, an incredible state of mixed media substance has been digitalized and their duplication made simple with no markdown in astounding through every crime and unapproved conveyance channels. Consumer-degree confirmation with utilizing present day-to-day gear, additionally will expand the consciousness of the issue of illegal exchange and is as of now utilized in different regions. In option, data created because of code assertion can be utilized by the item proprietor to examine areas wherein fake items are provided, which incorporates the likelihood of distinguishing resistant inventory network operators.

There are numerous prevalent innovations that can be utilized by the buyer to capture whether or not the item is fake or genuine. Watermark is considered as identifiers, embedded in the first bundle image.[29] This is incredible pattern as of late and it is miles due to the blast level of class of bundling of the items is an extremely compelling methodology against duplicating which permit the following of the great inside the convey and dispersion chain.

The disadvantage of bundling is that things inside the bundle arrangement might be disposed from the pack and substituted with some other phenomenal. In this model, fixing ought is done to alleviate this risk. To be utilized as a method for copyright security, advanced watermark is implanting concealed measurements into the bundle that cannot be changed and it acknowledges the quality of the product.[28] The human eye is capable to identify the adjustments to the lower regularities. So it is miles higher to embed a watermark into a picture[2] by method for altering colossal detail factors of its multiresolution demonstration. In this chapter, first we make a database at that point and train it for highlighting extraction. After that we proposed a calculation to accommodate whether an item is fake or not. Duplicate medicine is very risky to our health, such as duplicates of "Divine Noni Gold".[32] It assists to increase the human body's self-healing mechanism.[32]

It increases digestive quality in the body and benefits in sugar control in blood and has the cholesterol dropping mechanisms, and it also aids to protect the nervous system and in cancer detection. When intruders alter ingredients of medicine then it is very harmful to user's health. Nowadays, there are various types of Noni products found in the market. Thus, to preserve the originality of the medicine, we have to build a mobile application, and when we are purchasing medicine, first click the photo of the product,, and by using this application through Internet, we will be able to detect duplicate medicine.

2.5.5 BRAIN-TUMOR DETECTION

Cerebrum tumor recognition is a functioning territory of research in mind picture preparing. Here, a system is recommended to the section and arrange the brain tumor utilizing attractive reverberation pictures (MRI). Deep neural networks–based design is utilized for tumor or cell division. Here, multiple layers are utilized that comprise convolutional, ReLU, and a softmax layers. The information MRI picture is isolated into various fixes, and afterward the inside pixel estimation of every fix is provided to the deep neural network. It dole out marks as per focus pixels and perform division. A standout among the most loathsome sorts of unwanted cell division is known as harmful cell division or tumors.[31] Gliomas and lymphomas are the well-known harmful tumor.

Gliomas incorporate subsections of essential unwanted cell growth which degree from second rate to progressively infiltrative dangerous tumors. They have greatest pervasiveness with exceptionally great death rate. They are categorized into high-grade glioma (HGG) and low-grade glioma (LGG). HGG is low irruption and forceful when contrasted with the LGG. Patients of HGG as a rule do not endure more noteworthy than 1 year after the recognition procedure. We can use radiotherapy and chemotherapy for improvement in brain tumor. Ischemia stroke is the cerebrovascular contamination and normal intention of inability and passing around the world. The influenced cerebrum area (stroke sore) experiences numerous phases of the malady classified as subintense (23 h–2.5 weeks), interminable (>2.5 weeks), and intense (0–23 h). Segmentation[31] and ensuing quantitative sores appraisal in clinical pictures gives profitable information to the assessment of mind pathologies that are crucial for treatment arranging techniques, ailment checking forecast and movement of patient results. Moreover, careful wounds areas identify with explicit shortfalls relying upon influenced structure of the cerebrum.

The useful deficiencies delivered from wallop injury are connected with harm capacity to explicit cerebrum areas. At last, pathology outline in an exact manner is most essential advance in cerebrum tumor situation in which gauge of unwanted cell division amount of components area is required for further treatment arranging. Right division of the injury district in multidimensional pictures is progressively troublesome and testing work. The sore shows up in a heterogeneous manner, for example, more variety in size, area, recurrence, and shape makes it progressively hard to plan effective division stages. It is very unimportant to clarify wounds and drain's in components of cerebrum tumor, for example, the necrotic center and multiplied chambers. The apparently increasingly precise division results can be accomplished by the manual clarification through human specialists that is additionally tedious, costly, and dull undertaking. Besides, it is absolutely illogical if there should arise an occurrence of more investigations which presents extra bury spectator varieties. Increasingly effective robotized technique for tumor extraction is a noteworthy point in registering therapeutic pictures that gives independent and versatile strategies for qualitative assessment of unwanted cell growth. Brain stroke injuries have hyperserious advent and other white issue sores in groupings. Here it is generally difficult to accomplish factually earlier data identified with injury appearance and shape. Several administered strategies are utilized for cerebrum injuries division, for example, a popular classifier known as random forests classifier (RFC), strength-based highlights, and Gaussian mixture model.[31]

Logical and structural highlights are utilized for the identification of various sorts of cerebrum sores. Markov random field (MRF) is utilized for cerebrum injury division. The previously stated strategies are utilized with pointer made component removal strategy however the issues with pointer made technique are working out escalated when contrasted with profound learning strategies. At a similar time, profound learning strategies are all the more dominant when contrasted with managed techniques with the incredible capacity of model to adapt more separated highlights for assignment available. These highlights perform better just as they are precharacterized and carefully assembled capabilities. We can utilized convolutional neural networks (CNNs) to investigate the therapeutic imaging risky errands to accomplish best outcomes. Right off the bat, two-dimensional CNN can be utilized for sectioning neural films. Three dimensional mind division is acquired through preparing the two dimension cut independently. In spite of the basic engineering, better outcomes are accomplished by utilizing these methods showing CNN potential. Huge assortment of parameters increasingly adaptive power and huge recollection necessities are required completely in CNN model. Patches are extricated from multiscale figures and then joined into multiple patches to evade the completely CNN systems. Real cause is disheartening the CNN use since it has moderate derivation to adaptively progressive cost. Subsequently, classifier predispositions into uncommon classes may result in cell division. A CNN prototype is intended to prepare tests through circulation of parts that are near genuine parts; however, oversectioned pixels focus toward off base grouping in primary stage. Next preparing stage is likewise exhibited, in which fixes on separation parts are consistently extricated from info picture. Two periods of preparing arrangement may be inclined to overfitting and furthermore increasingly sensitive to first classifier system. At that point, thick preparing technique is utilized for system preparing. This strategy presented lopsidedness class mark that is like uniform examining. Weight cost work is utilized to beat this issue. Manual change of system affectability is given yet it turns out to be progressively hard to deal with multiclass issues by utilizing this strategy. The general article association is as per the following: characterizes related work. Nitty-gritty exhibited proposed steps are referenced here. Then deep neural network results are depicted in this section. At last the end of this exploration work is outlined in various procedures.

 Unwanted cell mass impact can be estimated by the injury development structures. The voxels gives accommodating data used to getting flatter divisions outcomes by the MRF.[20] MRF strategy is utilized for mind tumor cell division. Generative models well sum up shrouded information[8] with certain constraints at the preparation system. These strategies can gain proficiency with the example of mind tumor without using a particular model. These kinds of techniques for the most part consider indistinguishable and autonomous voxels circulation through setting highlights data. Because of this cause, disengaged groups of voxels might be segregated erroneously in the off base parts, now and then in anatomically and physiological impossible areas.

To maintain a strategic distance from these issues, numerous scientists included neighborhood data through installing probabilistic expectations into a random field (RF) classifier. Profound CNN models are utilized to automatically learn chains of importance of information highlights. CNN can keep running over patches by utilizing the bit trap. In cell division, ongoing techniques are using neural network. Three-dimensional channels can take benefits over the MR nature; however, adaptive burden is elevated. Double CNN is utilized to distinguish the total tumor area. At that point cells are connected to soft division outcomes before the CNN performs multiclass segregation between the tumor districts (Figures 2.8 and 2.9).

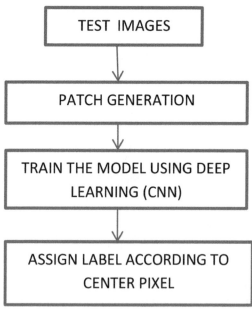

FIGURE 2.8 Brain-tumor detection using convolution neural network.

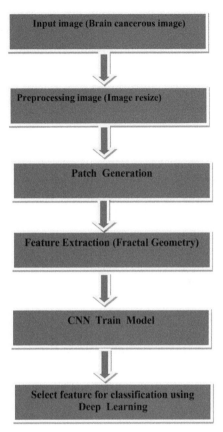

FIGURE 2.9 Brief procedure of brain-tumor detection using CNN.

CNN is prepared on separated fixes in every voxel plane, and yields of last layer, softmax and random forest (RF) are utilized to prepare the model. Cerebrum cell division method is isolated into parallel assignments and proposed organized expectations based on CNN as an initial learning model. Marks of patches are assembled into groups and neural network predicts input participation on every bunch. CNN are utilized for the removal in MR pictures. It is utilized to accomplish further CNN model. We demonstrate the concise synopsis of existing techniques.

Real commitment of this critique is as per the following:

1. Modified deep neural network model depends on multilayers subsequently proficiently portioning the cerebrum cell mass.

2. Info MRI picture is isolated into different patches and afterward focus pictorial element mark of each fix is determined and provided to the DNN which recovers the aftereffects of division just as grouping.
3. Accomplished outcomes are assessed with late strategies which demonstrate that DNN model performed superior to existing procedures.

Nowadays, it is very important to predict brain tumor and the category it belongs. It is very crucial part that how can an illiterate people be able to know whether he suffering from tumor or not. But it is possible in IoT. In present age, everyone can use hand-held devices called mobile phones. By using IoT and with the proper technology, we will be able to build an app. By using that application in mobiles, a person will be able to predict whether they are suffering from tumor or not. It is a cost-effective and simple technique to predict cancer.

2.6 CONCLUSION

The utilization of IoT is extending well in each part of the social protection system. Here, we have investigated various uses of IoT in various uprights of the helpful business. Initiating from the drug watching and the administrators, digitization of facilities to telemedicine care, we examined each feasible region at which IoT advancement can improve the procedures. Compelling the quick elevating of human administrations costs while extending restorative and inclusive incorporation to all—the fundamental goals of therapeutic administrations change—will require essential upgrades in the introduction of our structure for social protection. We set forward the leading body of trustees' assessment that the focal targets of switch are to carry on and improve prosperity and flourishing, to make fundamental prosperity consideration general, and to help the capable use of obliged resources. The past zones of this record have given a broad structure to assessing whether and how novel change suggestions would look for after these destinations. The parts of that structure—extending access to social protection, containing restorative administrations costs, ensuring nature of thought, financing change, and improving the system for convincing change—all ought to be tended to if structure execution is really to be improved. A whole deal perspective is essential.

A framework for reviewing change, for instance, that we have suggested, will be useful both for the basic evaluation of recommendation and for the examination of progression after some time. No ifs, ands or buts, to be most significant, as the outcomes of progress attempts spread out the warning gathering's recommendations should be at risk to a comparable kind of constant appraisal as the progressions themselves. The unconventionality of the restorative administrations structure—and of prosperity itself—shows genuine troubles to change, and these challenges are increased by the various critical and every now and again engaging interests that have a stake in both the extensive ways and confounded nuances of course of action change. Change recommendation that consideration on a very basic level on cash related issues and destinations without seeing that improved introduction requires basic changes in how therapeutic administrations is dealt with and gave are presumably not going to achieve the goals outlined here. Change recommendation must demonstrate their general method to manage request, for instance, how social protection specialists are to be appropriately arranged and passed on (tallying foreseen that responses ought to promote signals from refreshed helpers), how superior information is to be arranged to progress implementation, and how nature of thought can be kept up and improved inside resource prerequisites. Finally, the difference in our therapeutic administrations system should be grasped in a comparative soul of incessant improvement and reclamation that has so consistently been the foundation of achievement in America. The noteworthy changes required for feasible change, despite when the nation develops the present characteristics of its human administrations structure, demand that we gain for a reality. To do that we need incredible information and sound examinations of results, versatility, and imagination in responding to that information, and a withstanding base on the stresses of the all-inclusive community, the prosperity and success of which we hope to improve. It is hard to anticipate where IoT restorative devices are rushing toward—anyway we are certain that with the rising in eagerness for IoT and the money being spent in social protection advancements, valuable things will without a doubt happen in this space.

KEYWORDS

- IoT
- Cloud
- WBAN
- QoS
- GPS
- MAC
- TDMA

REFERENCES

1. Buckley, J. *From RFID to the Internet of Things: Pervasive Networked Systems*; Report on the Conference Organized by DG Information Society and Media, Networks and Communication Technologies Directorate, Brussels, March 6–7, 2006.
2. Chui, M.; Löffler, M; Roberts, R. The Internet of Things. http://tc.indymedia.org/files/bigbrother/internet-spy-all.pdf.
3. Complete RFID Analysis and Forecasts, 2008–2018. www.idtechex.com/research-reports/.
4. Kriplean, T. et al. Physical Access Control for Captured RFID Data. *IEEE Pervasive Comput.* **2007,** *6* (4), 48–55.
5. Hong, W. Key Technology of Telemedicine Based on 3G Network. *Chin. Hosp.* **2010,** *14* (7), 47–50.
6. Xu, R.; Xu, Z. T.; Li, L. B. Scheduling Solving of Telemedicine System in Multi-Expert Diagnosis. *Appl. Res. Comput.* **2020,** *27* (9), 3553–3555.
7. Fen-huaa, W.; Xina, N.; Guo-lianga, H.; Zhi-lianga, W. Application of Network of Things Technology on System of Status Detector. *Appl. Res. Comput.* **2010,** *27* (9), 3375–3380.
8. Li, W.; Yue, Z.; Long-fei, Z. ECG Data Processing Mechanism of Remote Wireless ECG Monitor. *Comput. Eng.* **2010,** *36* (15), 291–293.
9. Sosa, J.; Bowman, H.; Tielsch, J.; Powe, N.; Gordon, T.; Udelsman, R. The Importance of Surgeon Experience for Clinical and Economic Outcomes from Thyroidectomy. *Ann. Surg.* **1998,** *228* (3), 320330.
10. Sung, W.; Chiang, Y. Improved Particle Swarm Optimization Algorithm for Android Medical Care IoT Using Modified Parameters. *J. Med. Syst.* **2012,** *36* (6), 3755–3763.
11. Hassanalieragh, M.; Page, A.; Soyata, T.; Sharma, G.; Aktas, M.; Mateos, G.; Kantarci, B.; Andreescu, S. Health Monitoring and Management Using Internet of Things (IoT)

Sensing with Cloud Based Processing: Opportunities and Challenges. *IEEE Xplore* **2015**, 285291.
12. Takacs, J.; Pollock, C.; Guenther, J.; Bahar, M.; Napier, C.; Hunt, M. Validation of the Fitbit One Activity Monitor Device During Treadmill Walking. *J. Sci. Med. Sport* **2014**, *17* (5), 496500.
13. Fuentes, M.; Vivar, M.; Burgos, J.; Aguilera, J.; Vacas, J. Design of an Accurate, Low Cost Autonomous Data Logger for PV System Monitoring Using Arduino™ That Complies with IEC Standards. *ScienceDirect* **2014**, *130*, 529543.
14. Bauer, H.; Patel, M.; Veira, J. The Internet of Things: Sizing Up the Opportunity, 2014. http://www.mckinsey.com/industries/hightech/ourinsights/theinternetofthingssizing uptheopportunity.
15. Moorthy, K.; Munz, Y.; Sarker, S.; Darzi, A. Objective Assessment of Technical Skills in Surgery. *BMJ* **2014**, *327*, 10321037.
16. Kanis, J. *Assessment of Osteoporosis at the Primary Healthcare Level*; WHO Scientific Group Technical Report; The University of Sheffield, 2007; p 1339.
17. Hak, D.; Wu, H.; Dou, C.; Mauffrey, C.; Stahel, P. Challenges in Subtrochanteric Femur Fracture Management. *Orthopedics* **2015**, *38* (8), 498502.
18. Wani, M.; Wani, M.; Sultan, A.; Dar, T. Subtrochanteric Fractures: Current Management Options. *Internet J. Orthop. Surg.* **2009**, *17* (2), 18. https://print.ispub.com/api/0/ispubarticle/8827.
19. *LCP Proximal Femoral Plate 4.5/5.0 Surgical Technique*; DePuy Synthes, 2015; p 132.
20. *LCP Distal Femur Plate 4.5/5.0*; DePuy Synthes, 2007; p 18.
21. Leunig, M.; Hertel, R. Thermal Necrosis after Tibial Reaming for Intramedullary Nail Fixation. *J. Bone Joint Surg.* **1996**, *78B* (4), 584587.
22. Kim, S. J.; Yoo, J.; Kim, Y. S.; Shin, S. W. Temperature Change in Pig Rib Bone During Implant Site Preparation by Low Speed Drilling. *J. Appl. Oral Sci.* **2010**, *18* (5), 522527.
23. Reodique, A. *Noise Considerations for Integrated Pressure Sensors*; NdXPFreescale Semiconductor, volume AN1646, 2005; pp 17.
24. Alper, B.; Hand, J.; Elliott, S.; Kinkade, S.; Hauan, M.; Onion, D.; Sklar, B. How Much Effort is Needed to Keep Up with the Literature Relevant for Primary Care? *J. Med. Lib Assoc.* **2004**, *92* (4), 429437.
25. Bertollo, N.; Walsh, W. R. Drilling of Bone: Practicality, Limitations and Complications Associated with Surgical Drill Bits. In *Biomechanics in Applications;* Klika, V., Ed.; 2011. ISBN: 9789533079691.
26. Augustin, G.; Zigman, T.; Davila, S.; Udiljak, T.; Staroveski, T.; Brezak, D.; Babic, S. Cortical Bone Drilling and Thermal Osteonecrosis. *Clin. Biomech.* **2011**, *27* (4), 313325.
27. Chitkara, R.; Ballhaus, W.; Acker, O.; Song, B.; Sundaram, A.; Popova, M. *The Internet of Things: The Next Growth Engine for the Semiconductor Industry*; PwC, 2015; 136.
28. Gonzalez, R. C.; Woods, R. E. *Digital Image Processing*, 2nd ed.; Pearson International Edition: London.
29. Najafi, E. A Robust Embedding and Blind Extraction of Image Watermarking Based on Discrete Wavelet Transform. *Depart. Math. Faculty Sci., Urmia Univ. Iran Springer Math. Sci.* **2017**, *11*, 307–318. DOI: 10.1007/s40096-017-0233-1.

30. Bezdek, J. C. *Pattern Recognition with Fuzzy Objective Function Algorithms*; Springer Science & Business Media, 2013.
31. Corso, J. J; Sharon, E. Efficient Multilevel Brain Tumor Segmentation with Integrated Bayesian Model Classification. *IEEE Trans. Med. Imaging* **2008,** *27* (5).
32. Buyya, R.; Vecchiola, C.; Thamaraiselvi, S. *Mastering Cloud Computing*; McGraw Hill.

CHAPTER 3

ANALYSIS OF EFFICIENCIES BETWEEN EEG AND MRI: A SURVEY

NAMRATA P. MOHANTY[1*], SWETA SHREE DASH[1], and TRIPTI SWARNKAR[2]

[1]Department of Computer Science & Engineering

[2]Department of Computer Application, ITER, S'O'A University, Bhubaneswar, Odisha

*Corresponding author. E-mail: namratam54@gmail.com

ABSTRACT

There is no doubt that depression is spreading its influence all over the globe starting from teenagers to adults. No one in today's world is free from its clutches. Human–machine interaction that is a part of artificial intelligence has paved its path in detecting this terrible disorder before the onset of its severity. With the help of machine learning (ML) and Internet of things (IoT), the IoT is closely associated with cyber–physical interaction for real-time data processing, providing quick analysis of the brain signals whereas ML helps classify the unknown samples by learning from the known ones, predicting depression in individuals from a much earlier time. In this chapter, we have made a survey of various research work done on electroencephalography (EEG) signals, magnetic resonance imaging (MRI) scans, and various techniques and ML approaches used by them in the detection of depression. The chapter also presents a survey on the number of papers published per year based on both the EEG and MRI reports. Our survey suggested that although a lot more papers have been published on MRI reports for depression prediction, EEG still holds its place due to its pocket-friendly, noninvasive and time-effective factors of accurately detecting the brain's electrical activity within a short span. We have also found out that there is a need of discovering more effective ML techniques for real-time data acquisition and classification for an improved detection of depression in the earliest possible time. In this chapter, we have also tried to demonstrate various IoT–ML-related works that help the society in predicting depression and related seizures, trauma, and injuries occurring within the brain much more effectively in the earliest possible time.

3.1 INTRODUCTION

Persistent feeling of sadness or worthlessness is termed depression[99] and can even lead to suicide in extreme cases.[1] According to a survey taken by the World Health Organization, almost 350 million people all over the globe are suffering from depression[1]. Hence, we can correctly say that it is one of the leading contributors to the burden of diseases worldwide.[2,100]

Till date, there are no effective prediction techniques, nor any physiological measurements or biological markers to diagnose depression at an early stage.[2]

There exist several types of depression such as bipolar disorder,[67] melancholic depression, seasonal affective disorder, and dysthymic disorder.[3,39]

The symptoms usually include a loss of interest in activities previously enjoyed, insomnia, fatigue, feeling of worthlessness or guilt, and impaired ability to concentrate or make decisions. To our surprise, even sleep disturbances can lead to depression in adults leading to more serious comorbidities.[53]

Depression—more particularly called MDD, that is, major depressive disorder[71]—has several causative factors happening all around us, which makes the prediction and detection process of depression more complicated. Depression is not any particular disease, rather it is the main cause of disability worldwide. It is not just a simple disease, rather it is the root cause of many other terrible diseases such as schizophrenia, dementia, even strokes, osteoarthritis, diabetes, and cancers.

Manifestation of depression is strongly influenced by various factors such as psychological, social, and biochemical ones. Not only these, but also there are a lot of other factors responsible for the same, due to which the challenges we face in this field are vast. We need to analyze each and every aspect of depression, both the internal factors and the external ones,

Analysis of Efficiencies between EEG and MRI

with utmost care. It is distributed across networks in the brain, and varieties of depression can be present in various neural networks. Prior to the onset of depression, its symptoms can show up in any internal portion of the human body: physiological changes in the brain, imbalances in the body, etc. As depression is not any particular disease, predicting it has become one of the most difficult challenges in the field of medical science. Though machine learning (ML) techniques have been used to predict depression by taking into account various symptoms and psychological factors, we still never know from and in which way depression can show up. Mostly, there are two important means of taking the recordings of the brain waves: electroencephalography (EEG) and magnetic resonance imaging (MRI). EEG records the brain's electrical activity over a period of 10–15 s. Figure 3.1 shows a sample recording of the EEG signal over a period of 60 s. MRI captures the detailed image of the brain and brainstem using magnetic field and radio waves. Along with that, the brain–computer interface (BCI) is gaining popularity nowadays due to its widespread connectivity, cheaper price, and real-time data streaming and processing, providing much more efficient outcomes.

Till date, there have been more than 5 lakh papers published on depression, using both the fMRI and EEG signals and the number of publications that are increasing every year over the past decade. Figure 3.1 shows the number of publications based on EEG signal analysis only whereas Figure 3.2 shows a comparison between the number of papers published on the basis of EEG signals and MRI scans between 1950 and 2018.

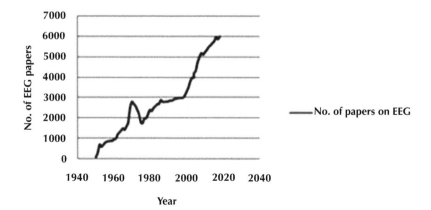

FIGURE 3.1 Number of EEG papers.

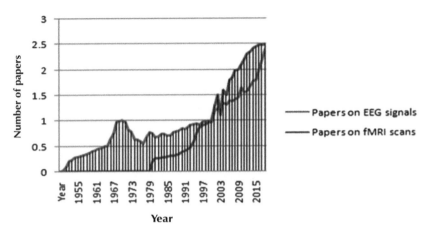

FIGURE 3.2 Number of both EEG and fMRI papers.

From 2001 onward, there have been vigorous studies on both fMRI and EEG signals, due to which there can be a strong comparison and critical analysis in the performance accuracy of prediction of depression of both fMRI scans and EEG signals. This analysis uses the papers from 2001 onward for the purpose of our survey.

3.2 CRITICAL REVIEW OF THE LITERATURES

In our research work, we have reviewed various papers on depression by taking both the EEG datasets and the MRI scanning reports. We have discussed the contribution of various ML techniques in the prediction of depression as well as the relationship between depression and seizure formation. We have also put forward some of the important points of why EEG signals are more efficient in the prediction of depression than the MRI scans.

3.2.1 DISCUSSION

From the previous critical survey, we have found out three major challenges in this field of diagnosing depression using ML. Those are

- seizure formation and depression,
- depression and ML, and
- EEG vs. MRI.

Dataset used EEG recordings

Author	Dataset	Objective/work done	Performance measures	Findings	Observation
Knott et al.[9]	EEG signal Obtained from the patients of the American Psychiatric Association, 1994	Classification	Accuracy	Efficiently classified 91.3% of patients and controls	It is one among those few examinations that inspects a moderately extensive variety of frightfully and factually determines EEG includes in connection to clinical wretchedness and they have acquired an exactness of 91.3%
Fan et al.[31]	EEG signals Shanghai Mental Health Center	Classification Algorithm-Backpropagation algorithm	Accuracy	Obtained an accuracy of 60%	Successful differentiation among the three types of subjects, that is, normal subjects, schizophrenic patients and the depressed ones has been performed using back propagation neural network algorithm
Li and Fan[32]	EEG signals	Classification Algorithm- BpNN, ANN, SOM	Accuracy	Obtained an accuracy between 60 and 80% for BPNN and 40 and 60% for SOM	In this paper, they have successfully distinguished among the three types of subjects, that is, normal subjects, schizophrenic patients, and the depressed ones using two ANN approaches, which are BPNN and self-organizing competitive neural network
Chisci et al.[18]	EEG signals Freiburg database	Classification Classifiers-SVM	Sensitivity	Obtained a sensitivity of 100% in their experiment	By using computer aided prediction algorithm, an automated seizure-prediction system has been proposed

Dataset used EEG recordings (*Continued*)

Author	Dataset	Objective/work done	Performance measures	Findings	Observation
Li et al.[6]	EEG signal Recorded by EEG system, Model LQWY-N, Sunray, China	Classification	Accuracy	Obtained an accuracy of 80% by correctly classifying 14 out of 20 controls. Also obtained specificity of 70% and sensitivity of 90% by classifying 18 out of 20 controls	In this, they have confirmed that wavelength entropy is an effective and efficient method of studying the EEG activity because of its capability of processing short and nonstationery signals like EEG epochs
Hosseinifard et al.[10]	EEG signal Atieh Psychiatry Centre	Linear and nonlinear features extraction, Classification Classifiers: kNN, LDA, LR Algorithm: Genetic algorithm	Accuracy	The author has found out effective classification methods to predict depression with an accuracy of 90%	Here various features have been extracted various linear and nonlinear features and showed how they can be helpful in predicting depression with maximum accuracy which can be helpful to assist psychiatrist in future as well
Williamson et al.[19]	EEG signals Freiburg database	Classification SVM classifier	Accuracy	Obtained an accuracy of 85.54%	An automated seizure prediction model has been using computer aided algorithm
Gadhoumi et al.[27]	EEG signal Freiberg database	Signal analysis using continuous wavelet transformation	Sensitivity and specificity	Seizure prediction model with sensitivity of less than 85%	An automated seizure-prediction technique has been proposed with a sensitivity of less than 85%
Ghaderyan et al.[21]	EEG signals Freiburg database	Classification Classifier-SVM, kNN	Sensitivity	Seizure prediction model with a sensitivity of 98%	A mechanized seizure-forecast framework has been proposed which can additionally diminish computational multifaceted nature, that is, its complexity

Analysis of Efficiencies between EEG and MRI

Dataset used EEG recordings *(Continued)*

Author	Dataset	Objective/work done	Performance measures	Findings	Observation
Fujiwara et al.[23]	EEG dataset Freiburg database	Feature extraction, Analysis of variability signals from the heart rate	Accuracy	Presented a successful seizure prediction model with sensitivity of 99.8%	Based on the analysis of variability signals from heart rate they have proposed an ideal seizure prediction technique, in their experiment
Zhang et al.[25]	EEG signal Freiburg database	Differential equation-based mathematical model	Accuracy	Proposed a seizure prediction model with sensitivity of 100%	They have developed a model for quantifying the dynamic advancement of EEG signals amid seizure development
Gautam et al.[7]	EEG signals Recorded from the residents of Lucknow using the bio semi tool[66]	Feature extraction, Classification Classifiers: kNN, regression tree	Accuracy	From the whole experiment of predicting depression, they have concluded that women are more depressed than men	The primary aim of this experiment is to predict the level of depression among people belonging to both urban and rural regions, which has been successfully predicted by using different machine learning techniques through MATLAB. This study is basically a region-based survey where samples of EEG signals have been collected from the people residing in the Lucknow city of India
Subhani et al.[54]	EEG signals	Classification, Classifiers: LR, SVM, Naive Bayes classifier	Accuracy, specificity, and sensitivity	They have obtained 94.6% accuracy for a2-level identification of stress and 83.4% for multilevel identification of stress	The main contribution of this chapter is to develop an experimental paradigm for inducing stress at multiple levels and to provide a framework for EEG data analysis to identify pressures at multiple levels

Dataset used EEG recordings *(Continued)*

Author	Dataset	Objective/work done	Performance measures	Findings	Observation
Vuckovic et al.[4]	EEG signal http://kdd.ics.uci.edu/ database	Classification Classifiers used: ANN, SVM, LDA	Accuracy, sensitivity, and specificity	In the experiment they have obtained an accuracy of 90%	Here, it has been shown that the accuracy of LDA is as close as ANN due to its simple structure and the specificity and sensitivity were also higher showing that they are not biased toward false positives and false negatives
Prasad et al.[5]	EEG signal Recorded by the BrainMarker, model: DEV12001EE	Classification Classifiers used: SVM, kNN, SSD (Subspace discriminant)	Accuracy	In their experiment they have obtained an accuracy of 70% in the sentiment analysis of the depressed patients	Machine learning techniques of EEG signals along with suicidal notes can be of great help in detecting suicidal ideation and indirect sensing of sentiments
Breda et al.[29]	Blended treatment (BT) dataset, treatment as usual (TAU) dataset	Classification, Classifiers-Random forest, kNN	ROC curve	Their outcomes recommended that significant prescient power is available in the pattern dataset and they have effectively anticipated TAU and BT treatments with AUC esteems somewhere in the range of 0.71 and 0.78 on an autonomous test set	The capability of foreseeing treatment accomplishment for patients in psychological wellness care has been investigated, which can inevitably improve the way toward coordinating effective treatment types to individuals
Acharya et al.[33]	EEG signals	Classification of a 13-layer deep convolution neural network model	Accuracy, specificity, and sensitivity	Obtained 93.54% accuracy using the left hemisphere EEG data and 95.49% accuracy from the right hemisphere EEG data	Abnormal early dynamic individual pattern of functional network in low gamma band has been found out, which is useful for depression recognition

Dataset used EEG recordings *(Continued)*

Author	Dataset	Objective/work done	Performance measures	Findings	Observation
Dataset used: MRI Scannings					
Gong et al.[12]	MRI scans obtained from people of Han, China who were previously diagnosed with depression and records were also taken from healthy subjects with no history of depression	Image processing, Classification Classifier: SVM	Accuracy	Accuracy obtained is 67.39% for RDD and 76.09% for NDD	In this study it has been found out that the gray matter and white matter have diagnostic and prognostic potential in the prediction of depression
Wise et al.[11]	MRI scanning reports, Positron emission tomography reports	Image processing and pattern recognition	Accuracy	They concluded that functional and structural changes in the mood-regulating system may be used as diagnostic biomarkers for depression, and they also reviewed fMRI studies showing differences in ACC effects and predicting responses to pharmacological and psychological treatments	Several papers on predicting depression in different types of brain scans using image processing and various machine learning techniques have been reviewed and attention has been paid to the fact that neuroimaging potential becomes part of clinical equipment and can improve diagnostic accuracy in prediction. Depression is in the near future
Meng et al.[14]	A total of 50 healthy control and 47 schizophrenia patients sMRI, f	Regression	Accuracy	They have found out that as compared to a single modality, multimodal combination achieves higher prediction	Their work features the potential utility of multimodal brain-imaging biomarkers to eventually inform clinical depression making

Dataset used EEG recordings (*Continued*)

Author	Dataset	Objective/work done	Performance measures	Findings	Observation
	MRI, DTI (fractional anisotrophy)			accuracy and enables individualized prediction on multiple clinical measures to be more efficient	
Pyeong et al.[13]	Retrospective dataset of 76 patients obtained after CAS	Classification Classifiers: ANN, MLR Backpropagation algorithm using TensorFlow platform	ROC curve, accuracy	Obtained accuracy of 98.7% with 0.961 AUROC and the author has found out that ANN model is more powerful than MLR and SVM models in prediction of PHD	They have focused on the fact that prediction of hemodynamic depression after CAS is absolutely feasible in high-risk depressive patients using machine learning techniques such as ANN
Fonseka et al.[17]	MRI scans	Image processing, classification	ROC curve	They have summarized the data from studies, examining predictors of treatment response using structural and functional neuroimaging modalities, as they pertain to pharmacotherapy, psychotherapy, and stimulation treatment strategies	Focused on how neuroimaging biomarkers of the brain's structural and functional part may be useful in guiding treatment selection by prediction response and nonresponse outcomes
van der Burgh et al.[28]	MRI scans Obtained from patients of University Medical Centre Utrecht, the Netherlands	Image processing, Classification	Accuracy	Obtained an accuracy of 625%	Amyotrophic lateral sclerosis (ALS) is basically a neuromuscular disorder which usually happens with people suffering from dementia or stroke. It has a large variation in the

Dataset used EEG recordings *(Continued)*

Author	Dataset	Objective/work done	Performance measures	Findings	Observation
					survival rate. In this study they have efficiently evaluated the survival time of ALS patients on the basis of clinical characteristics with an accuracy of 62.5%
Schultz et al.[30]	fMRI scans	Classification	Accuracy	They have effectively predicted patients' reaction status with an exactness of up to 88.9% based on neuroimaging information utilizing SVM calculation	The capability of combining information from various neuroimaging modalities has been investigated to foresee treatment response in major depressive disorder

3.2.1.1 SEIZURE FORMATION AND DEPRESSION

Disorder in the nerve cell activity leading to the disturbances in the brain causing seizures or periods of unusual behavioral sensations or sometimes even a loss of awareness is referred to as "Epilepsy." Depression and seizure formation are like the two sides of the same coin. Most of the epileptic seizures are formed due to depression, which leads to a strong lifetime disability in the patients such as paralysis.

Individuals with depression or anxiety have been found to experience the ill effects of epilepsy more than those without depression or anxiety. Different cerebrum territories, including the frontal, temporal, and limbic regions, are associated with the biological pathogenesis of depression in individuals with epilepsy.[34] There are various studies on EEG signals using ML techniques to predict epilepsy.[86] ML techniques are of great help for the detection of epilepsy from the analysis of EEG signals.[94]

In 2018, Acharya et al. have focused on seizure formation and prediction and how depression is related to seizure formation which is generally due to the sudden change in electrical activity of the brain.[35]

In 2009, Piotr Mirowski et al. have successfully investigated the efficiency of employing bivariate measures to predict seizures, occurring mostly by depression with a sensitivity of 71%.[36]

In 2017, Cho et al.[38] have concentrated on the proficiency of the phase lock value seizure forecast marker and have effectively predicted the seizure formation with an accuracy of 83.17%.

In 2017, Chu et al.[39] and Behnam et al.[92] have also investigated the prediction of seizure from the EEG signals of the depressed patients due to depression with a sensitivity of 86.67%. They have effectively dissected the signals to get access of the attractor state analysis to figure seizure arrangement from a lot of prior time.

In 2017, Zhang et al.[25] have analyzed the EEG signals and tried to develop a differential equation-based mathematical model for quantifying the dynamic advancements of the signals during the seizure formation.

In this paper, they have found that the synaptic plasticity has some major impact on the period of seizure formation.

In 2015, Faust et al.[37] reviewed the wavelet methodologies for computer-based seizure detection and epilepsy diagnosis with an accentuation on research revealed in the past decade.

Although both medical and psychobehavioral therapies have been found out for prediction and treatment that can ameliorate these conditions, but randomized trials are still needed for the confirmation of the same.[34]

3.2.1.2 DEPRESSION AND MACHINE LEARNING

Depression causes terrible havoc. If not predicted and controlled in time, it can eliminate the peace and happiness of a person's entire life. As science and technology advance, ML tools and techniques can easily predict depression from an earlier time, thereby maintaining this disability leading to disorders. ML describes a range of statistical techniques in which computer programs learn how to optimize the performance of classification or prediction tasks without explicit parameterization.[96] ML algorithms typically learn, extract, identify, and map underlying patterns to unrestrictedly identify groups of depressed individuals.[41] There are many classifiers and prediction algorithms that not only detect depression but also detect several serious diseases with the highest accuracy.[42] ML also helps us to improve the diagnosis and prognosis of bipolar depression.

In 2017, Dipnal et al. have taken 96 "lifestyle environ" variables from National Health and Nutrition Examination department and supported the use of unsupervised GLUMM to form ordered depressive clusters from multitudinous lifestyle variables to better explore the heterogeneous mental health problems with the potential to unearth cover results.

There are two methods we can use to predict depression: by analyzing the EEG signals and MRI scanning reports and image processing. The authors of Ref. [43] have analyzed different prediction algorithms and different methods for image processing for the detection of depression even before the individual comes to know that he/she is suffering from depression. They have also focused on different risk factors leading to depression and have also concluded that ML techniques can predict depression much earlier.

In 2001, Ahearn et al.[15] had taken MRI scans of 20 depressed subjects, and by performing image processing and classification, they found that people with abnormal MRI findings are more inclined toward mood disorders as well as suicide. The goal of this study was to compare MRI findings in unipolar patients and without a history of suicide attempts, they have discovered that unipolar patients with a background marked by a history of suicide attempts exhibited essentially more subcortical gray matter hyperintensities compared with patients without such a history.

Khanna et al.[44] have focused on the effect of respiratory depression in extremely low acuity hospital conditions by seeking answers from initial trials where they have tried to derive a risk prediction score for respiratory depression on patients around the globe.

In 2016, Gifford et al.[45] have presented a review paper that focuses on the potential for neuroimaging measures to facilitate prediction of the onset of MDD.

In 2018, Karim et al.[46] have analyzed MRI scannings and performed image processing and logistic classification in late life depression prediction with a sensitivity and specificity of 72 and 68%, respectively. Here, they have efficiently proposed a method of predicting treatment response in late night depression by utilizing the functional imaging metrics in response to a single dose of a pharmacological intervention.

In 2017, Kim et al.[47] have also analyzed the MRI scans and performed pattern recognition, image processing, and classification using SVM classifiers and have obtained an accuracy of 89%. In this paper, they have successfully proved that the concept of combining multicenter MRI data to create a single, well-performing model is absolutely possible.

Sato et al.,[48] in their experiment, for the very first time, have used the ML techniques to distinguish remitted major depressed from control participants with 78.3% accuracy using a recently identified neural signature of guilt-selective function disconnection.

ML techniques consist of various methodologies that are helpful in developing prediction models from empirical data to make accurate prediction on current data.[49] Then validation measures are used to access how well a model developed by the learning method will perform on new unseen data.

In their paper, Alghwiri et al.[52] studied the relationship between depression and balance disorders in patients with multiple sclerosis (MS) in 2018. In this study, they found that balance disorders and depressive symptoms are often associated with people having MS.

Larger studies state that depression, termed a severe illness, has a lifetime prevalence of between 10 and 20%.[51] It is one of the most important factors, even for suicide that accounts for around 15% among the depressed controls.[61] The majority of depressed cases were undiagnosed. It can be one among many, starting from a simple skin disease to cancers and strokes as well.

Depression is such a phenomenon that is poorly understood but clinically very crucible.[50] Depression can give rise to memory disruption, which can lead to several other major disability causing issues. Dhillon et al. in 2018 have reviewed several neuroscientific research to stimulate the impact of depression on memory. The more we understand the mechanism, the more we can alter the mechanism to stop disruption occurring from depression.

In 2018, Casanova et al.[55] examined the feasibility of evaluating an anatomical index that can be utilized as an Alzheimer's disease risk factor in women's health activity MRI study using MRI data. They have taken a well-characterized database, that is, Alzheimer's disease neuroimaging database and by using neuroimaging methods and high-dimensional classifiers have calculated the cognitive scores. The scores indicated a relationship with intellectual weakness, psychological capacity, subjective status, and so forth. Their work likewise gives extra help to the utility of artificial intelligence determined scores.

DeVille et al.[56] in 2018 compared introceptive and exteroceptive recall by implementing the introceptive and exteroceptive recall task among normal subjects and depressed patients and have found out that the introceptive cell is more associated with bilateral mid-to-posterior insula activation than exteroceptive cell. They have also shown that individuals with MDD exhibit decreased insula activity while recalling introceptic memories than normal subjects.

In 2018, the main objective of Dey et al.[57] was to find out whether decision-making is linked with depression or not. In their experiment, they have taken both high and low dysphoric individuals and engaged them in abstract thinking as well as concrete thinking followed by a writing task within a time period of 9 days. Later they have found out that in the case of depression, individuals take a longer duration in task competition but only in the case of abstract condition and not in the case of concrete condition. They have further stated that abstract thinking can contribute to more difficulties in depression whereas concrete thinking could reduce the same.

Palmwood et al.[58] in 2017 examined the potential deficits in three aspects, that is, conflict monitoring, conflict resolution, and overt behavioral inhibition with respect to the symptoms of depression. In their experiment, they have found that depression is related with impaired conflict resolution. ML is so well connected to depression that even the slightest onset of it can be detected by various ML techniques.

3.2.1.3 WHY EEG RATHER THAN MRI?

EEG signals refer to the recording of the brain's spontaneous electrical activity over a period of time while an MRI machine captures the detailed image of the brain and brain stem using magnetic field and radio waves.[35] For example, blood clots are mostly related to severe heart and kidney diseases. Taking images externally makes the prediction of the severity and the association of the clot with other organs difficult. But at the same time, if we can measure the flow of the liquid over a particular period of time then it can be easily detected even from the initial stage just like the EEG signals. Though MRI scans are gaining popularity in the field of medical research, EEG has still not been completely replaced in the analysis of depression because of its noninvasive, economical, and easy operation factors.[101]

3.3 IoT–ML MODEL

Internet of things (IoT)—meaning the world to be connected to each other through cloud via Internet. IoT is gaining popularity and interest due to its ease of use, efficiency, and time-saving aspects. Real-time data processing and data streaming are the two main factors that are increasing the use of IoT in the field of medical science. The world of medical science is in strict need of real-time access to any sickness, injury or trauma occurring in the human body in order to provide them with the best treatment plan possible. Depression—a disorder that can lead to severe traumatic condition in the body needs real-time data access from the brain in order to predict it efficiently. Seizures occur time to time in the brain when the individual is in a state of severe depression, leading to the onset of stroke and thereby death (sometimes or leaving them physically handicapped). With the help of IoT, real-time data can be obtained from the brain for processing and ML helps in the analysis and the prediction of seizures at the same instant leading to the construction of a life-saving IoT–ML model. Researches are still continuing in this field to get a more efficient and ethical model that can even be used by the common man of the society.

Neurotechnology is the new field of medical science concentrating on the comprehension of the mind, cognizance, and perspectives and neural systems then again is the merger of this natural insight with machine knowledge for the most part alluding to the association between human cerebrum and hardware. In any case, the connection among neurotechnology and neural systems is extending far from one-directional action (cerebrum to the hardware system), toward bidirectional action. This takes into consideration messages to be sent from the PC straightforwardly to your cerebrum.

Neurotechnology is essentially using medical devices to track mind movement and screen its conduct. By utilizing electrical incitement and dissecting how the sensory system functions, scientists and doctors can gain insights in recognizing different ailments. The capacity to utilize brain signals and analyze a definite well-being appraisal can help distinguish different diseases, for example, Alzheimer's and mild cognitive impairment (MCI). Albeit a considerable lot of these advances are still in the trial stage, the impact that IoT has on social insurance cannot be disregarded and the potential outcomes are huge in joining technology as a key progression in the medical field.[114] Neurotechnology along with BCI is of great help when it comes to diagnosing any injuries occurring in the brain internally. Doctors along with scientists have been working for the integration of the most complex structure of the human body with computer-aided application for better time-saving instant-treatment plans.[110] With the growth of various aspects in the field of IoT, intense disability-causing disorders can be predicted to reduce the effect even before reaching the peak to give tremendous benefits. Researches are still there on how effective and ethical these integration processes can be in real-life scenarios.

In this paper, they have designed a BCI providing noninvasive signal recording,[109] minimum training, and a high information-transfer rate that can improve the performance of the system leading to better communication between the patients and the doctors' panels.

With the advancement in technologies, there are various equipment that can record the brain signals as well as take pictures of the complete brain and if this can be combined with the IoT providing real-time data processing and analysis then the accuracy of detecting any kind of seizures or trauma occurring within the brain, can promote to the next level, thereby helping the scientists and doctors in the treatment of the injuries in a much more efficient way.[105] In this paper they have proposed two real-time cognitive interaction applications, which are selective attention mechanism (SAM) and the long short-term memory (LSTM), where the former is used to distinguish between various features of the brain signals and the latter is used to distinguish interdimensional information obtained from SAM.

In most of the cases, the brain injuries that are diagnosed possess limited accuracy due to the lack of quantitative and delay in processing the data resulting in producing fewer effective results. In the paper,[103] they have proposed an IoT-based application system mostly targeting the athletes suffering from head injuries where they have designed a helmet that records the brain signals and seizures formed during the course of time and the frequency at which the seizures are changing, which enables the scientists and doctors to plan a more feasible treatment method that will ultimately lead to a successful cure, especially for the athletes within the minimum duration possible.

Yong et al.,[104] in their work, have developed an IoT neuroscience application where they have designed a multichannel, multisignal physiological sensing system that enables real-time processing of three types of data: EEG, electrocardiogram (ECG), and EMG, up to a period of 18 h and helps in better analysis by integrating the real-time streaming of data with the cloud enabling a complex and computationally intensive analytic system.[106,107]

IoT helps, not only in the field of data streaming and processing, but also in drug management and monitoring among the patients with severe illness. IoT with the help of radio frequency (RF) identification (RFIDs) has begun to find broader application in the field of medical material management visualization. It also helps in avoiding public health problems by aiding in the production, distribution, and tracking of medical devices and medicine. This increases the quality of medical treatment while reducing management costs. Research is continuing on a broader scale for integrating IoT in all the sectors of medical science starting from cardio department to the gynecic division. The concept of digital hospitals is coming into picture nowadays with the help of IoT, which can be of great help, especially to people belonging to the remotest areas of the society. The various aspects of digital hospitals can be broadly divided into patient information management, drug storage, medical emergency management, medical equipment and drug tracking, connected information sharing, and newborn anti-kidnapping system. Apart from this there are various other aspects such as data security related to broadcasting, data compression, and data storage which are being researched upon in order to get a completely well-structured and protected system for diagnosing a patient's health.

The IoT will reach and interface all parts of life. According to reports, by the end of 2020, over 200 billion gadgets will be assimilated, which equals 26 shrewd gadgets for each individual on Earth. The complete market capability of IoT innovation will reach up to 6.2 trillion USD with 38% of the all-out worth originating from gadgets in healthcare.[114] The development of Internet of Medical Things (IoMT) has allowed medical devices and applications to accumulate data as well as communicate with the healthcare IT systems via a wireless network.[114]

There is an increasing possibility for cell phones to discuss legitimately with IT frameworks through the technological advancements in consumer mobile devices, for example, RFID and near field communication. For the adult population of the society, rising healthcare costs and technological advancements have driven governments to present approaches concentrated on helping the IoMT area. With the expansion in the interest in the field of IoMT, biometric sensors have changed; how patients with long-haul ailments cooperate with their specialists. Regular checkups are no longer required as specialists can screen real-time data continuously and make recommendations as needed. This has resulted in the creation of a well-connected healthcare ecosystem with minimum pressure on hospital resources and more prominent adaptability and opportunity for patients.

Not only that but also the capacity to empower area following of patients and therapeutic gear utilizing sensor-based innovation have left the administration all alone, which in these days is alluded to as location-as-a-service. Pushing information into the cloud has just brought about the development of appropriate telemedicine, in the healthcare sector. Telemedicine carries adaptability to the very wild human services condition, starting from overseeing patients remotely to utilizing handheld gadgets to include patient subtleties and oversee the care. The treatment of different issues encompassing brain health is the key focus area for such applications and abilities. With the introduction of new technology, there is an enormous interest for consumer-based medical devices that are utilized to gather biometric data. The cases in which IoMT device can help vary from dependence suspension trackers to savvy thermometers, and monitoring frameworks for ECG testing. This takes into account that patient checking is to be effectively done remotely and gives experiences to medicinal service experts and the capacity to set alarms in the event of any spike or changes in the patients' conditions before it being fatal. One of the most recent achievements is the blaze glucose detecting gadget that enables you to check the blood glucose levels by examining a sensor worn on the patient's arm. This gadget will permit type 1 diabetes patients to deal with their condition while making their lives a lot simpler.[114]

In a report titled "2012–2020 Digital Brain Health Market," SharpBrains follows the advances of more than 50 organizations to provide robotic applications focused on brain function. In particular, these organizations offer web-based, versatile, and biometric solutions for investigating, screening, and improving cognitive and brain functions. In light of its findings, SharpBrains expects that by 2020, more than 1 million adults (only considering North America) will undergo annual brain health checks through their tablets. In addition, a subjective screening based on the iPad would suggest a higher number of diagnoses for Alzheimer's disease and MCI than neuroimaging. In any of the 10 countries, SharpBrains anticipate that patients with various sclerosis should begin to address their condition through a combination of online intelligence training and drug-based treatment.[113]

Cognitive testing on mobile phones will make it easier for athletes to analyze and monitor potential blackouts. Other brain applications focus on treating sleep disorders and depression through subjective treatment. For example, the report points out that the first brain-based biomarket will be approved by the FDA over the next 5 years to predict the response to depression treatment on an individual basis. Research and computerized mind instruments can ultimately help individuals improve their brain health in their daily lives. If a large system and associated advance payments are established to allow for the transmission, receipt, storage, and protection of these "big data," and this is only the beginning, then this medical advance must be completed immediately. The microwave and RF industry is the focus of this model. As an industry that is largely a communications and protection enterprise, whether it is for medical applications, a keen urban area, a brilliant family, or more, it can empower the IoT. This goal seems easy to achieve.[112,113] The IoT transforms our past simple business or protection applications into a broad approach in which everything is connected to machinery, business, consumers, and more.

3.4 CONCLUSION/FUTURE WORK

Depression is not as simple as it sounds like. More than just a disease, it can literally pose some serious challenges to the world of medical science in both accurate diagnosis and effective timely treatment. Apart from timely treatment, the most important factor in depression treatment is "predicting it" as no completely effective treatment has been found out yet. healthcare professionals need to understand the level of depression of the patients and the circumstances they are facing in their daily lives, which makes predicting the patient's risk of facing depression easier, and thereby providing the patients with an effective and a properly planned treatment. Many challenges still exist in the world of medical science regarding depression that ought to be researched thoroughly such as ultrafield MRI scanning in brainstem imaging, investigation of complex brain structure, acquisition of real-time data of both EEG signals and MRI scans, and data analysis using proper ML models. ML along with IoT has become an integral part of medical science, right from predicting the reason behind mild fever to the analysis of severe illness such as cancers and strokes. IoT plays an important role in directing the data and signals right away from the patient's body to the analysis system through cloud, which may be present at a greater distance. Forecasting information and data at the particular instant of the onset of the illness gives better opportunities to the doctors and scientists in analyzing and predicting it with greater accuracy when combined with the features of ML. Last but not the least, depression is something that should not be taken lightly and proper checkups by experienced professionals should be done in due time so as to get rid of this illness before the onset of its extreme phase.

KEYWORDS

- depression
- machine learning
- artificial intelligence
- EEG
- MRI

REFERENCES

1. Mallikarjun, H. M.; Suresh, H. N. Depression Level Prediction Using EEG Signal Processing. In *2014 International Conference on Contemporary Computing and Informatics (IC³I)*, Mysore, 2014; pp 928–933. DOI: 10.1109/IC3I.2014.7019674.
2. Liao, S.-C.; Wu, C.-T.; Huang, H.-C.; Cheng, W.-T.; Liu, Y.-H. Major Depression Detection from EEG Signals Using Kernel Eigen-Filter-Bank Common Spatial

Patterns. *Sensors (Basel)* **2017,** *17* (6), 1385. Published Online: Jun 14, 2017. DOI: 10.3390/s17061385.
3. Benazzi, F. Various Forms of Depression. *Dialogues Clin. Neurosci. J.* **2006,** *8* (2), 151–161.
4. Vuckovic, A.; Gallardo, V. J. F.; Jarjees, M.; Fraser, M.; Purcell, M. Prediction of Central Neuropathic Pain in Spinal Cord Injury Based on EEG Classifier. *Clin. Neurophysiol.* **2018,** *129* (8), 1605–1617. DOI: 10.1016/j.clinph.2018.04.750. Epub 2018 May 23.
5. Prasad, D. K.; Liu, S.; Chen, S.-H. A.; Quek, C. Sentiment Analysis Using EEG Activities for Suicidology. *Expert Syst. Appl.* **2018**. DOI: 10.1016/j.eswa.2018.03.011 (doc_10).
6. Li, Y.; Li, Y.; Tong, S.; Tang, Y.; Zhu, Y. More Normal EEGs of Depression Patients During Mental Arithmetic Than Rest. In *2007 Joint Meeting of the 6th International Symposium on Noninvasive Functional Source Imaging of the Brain and Heart and the International Conference on Functional Biomedical Imaging,* Hangzhou, 2007, pp 165–168. DOI: 10.1109/NFSI-ICFBI.2007.4387716 (doc_11).
7. Gautam, R.; Shimi, S. L. Features Extraction and Depression Level Prediction by Using EEG Signals. *Int. Res. J. Eng. Technol. (IRJET)* **2017,** *4* (5). (doc_12).
8. Ebrahimi, F; Mikaeili, M.; Estrada, E.; Nazeran, H. Automatic Sleep Stage Classification Based on EEG Signals by Using Neural Networks and Wavelet Packet Coefficients. In *30th Annual International IEEE EMBS Conference*, Vancouver, British Columbia, Canada, Aug 20–24, 2008; pp 1151–1154. DOI: 10.1109/IEMBS.2008.4649365. (doc_13).
9. Knott, V.; Mahoney, C.; Kennedy, S.; Evans, K. EEG Power, Frequency, Asymmetry and Coherence in Male Depression. *Psychiatry Res.: Neuroimaging Sect.* **2001,** *106*, 123–140. (doc_13).
10. Hosseinifard, B.; Moradi, M. H.; Rostami, R. Classifying Depression Patients and Normal Subjects Using Machine Learning Techniques. In *2011 19th Iranian Conference on Electrical Engineering*, Tehran, 2011; pp 1.
11. Wise, T.; Cleare, A. J.; Herane, A.; Young, A. H.; Arnone, D. Diagnostic and Therapeutic Utility of Neuroimaging in Depression: An Overview. *Neuropsychiatr. Dis. Treat.* **2014,** *10*, 1509–1522. DOI: 10.2147/NDT.S50156.
12. Gong, Q.; Wu, Q.; Scarpazza, C.; Lui, S.; Jia, Z.; Marquand, A.; Huang, X.; McGuire, P.; Mechelli, A. Prognostic Prediction of Therapeutic Response in Depression Using High-Field MR Imaging. *NeuroImage* **2011,** *55* (4), 1497–1503. DOI: 10.1016/j.neuroimage.2010.11.079.
13. Pyeong, J. J.; Chulho, K.; Byoung-Doo, O.; Jeong, K. S.; Yu-Seop, K. Prediction of Persistent Hemodynamic Depression after Carotid Angioplasty and Stenting using Artificial Neural Network Model. *Clin. Neurol. Neurosurg.* **2017**. https://doi.org/10.1016/j.clineuro.2017.12.005.
14. Meng, X.; Jiang, R.; Lin, D.; Bustillo, J.; Jones, T.; Chen, J.; Yu, Q.; Du, Y.; Zhang, Y.; Jiang, T.; Sui, J.; Calhoun, V. D. Predicting Individualized Clinical Measures by a Generalized Prediction Framework and Multimodal Fusion of MRI Data. *NeuroImage* **2016**. DOI: 10.1016/j.neuroimage.2016.05.026.
15. Ahearn, E. P.; Jamison, K. R.; Steffens, D. C.; Cassidy, F.; Provenzale, J. M.; Lehman, A.; Weisler, R. H.; Carroll, B. J.; Krishnan, K. R. MRI Correlates of Suicide Attempt History in Unipolar Depression. *Biol. Psychiatry* **2001,** *50* (4), 266–270.

16. Amoroso, N.; La Rocca, M.; Monaco, A.; Bellotti, R.; Tangaro, S. Complex Networks Reveal Early MRI Markers of Parkinson's Disease. *Med. Image Anal.* **2018**. DOI: 10.1016/j.media.2018.05.004.
17. Fonseka, T. M.; MacQueen, G. M.; Kennedy, S. H. Neuroimaging Biomarkers as Predictors of Treatment Outcome in Major Depressive Disorder. *J. Affect. Disord.* https://doi.org/10.1016/j.jad.2017.10.049.
18. Chisci, L.; Mavino, A.; Perferi, G.; Sciandrone, M.; Anile, C.; Colicchio, G.; Fuggetta, F. Real-Time Epileptic Seizure Prediction Using AR Models and Support Vector Machines. *IEEE Trans. Biomed. Eng.* **2010**, *57* (5), 1124–1132. DOI: 10.1109/TBME.2009.2038990. Epub 2010 Feb 17.
19. Williamson, J. R.; Bliss, D. W.; Browne, D. W.; Narayanan, J. T. Seizure Prediction Using EEG Spatiotemporal Correlation Structure. *Epilepsy Behav.* **2012**, *25* (2), 230–238. DOI: 10.1016/j.yebeh.2012.07.007. Epub 2012 Oct 2.
20. Zhang, Z.; Parhi, K. K. Low-Complexity Seizure Prediction from iEEG/sEEG Using Spectral Power and Ratios of Spectral Power. *IEEE Trans. Biomed. Circuits Syst.* **2016**, *10* (3), 693–706. DOI: 10.1109/TBCAS.2015.2477264.
21. Ghaderyan, P.; Abbasi, A.; Sedaaghi, M. H. An Efficient Seizure Prediction Method Using KNN-Based under Sampling and Linear Frequency Measures. *J. Neurosci. Methods*, **2014**, *232*, 134–142.
22. Vahabi, Z.; Amirfattahi, R.; Shayegh, F.; Ghassemi, F. Online Epileptic Seizure Prediction Using Wavelet-Based Bi-Phase Correlation of Electrical Signals Tomography. *Int. J. Neural Syst.* 2015, *25* (6), 1550028. DOI: 10.1142/S0129065715500288. Epub 2015 May 26.
23. Fujiwara, K.; Miyajima, M.; Yamakawa, T.; Abe, E.; Suzuki, Y.; Sawada, Y.; Kano, M.; Maehara, T.; Ohta, K.; Sasai-Sakuma, T.; Sasano, T.; Matsuura, M.; Matsushima, E. Epileptic Seizure Prediction Based on Multivariate Statistical Process Control of Heart Rate Variability Features. *IEEE Trans. Biomed. Eng.* **2016**, *63* (6), 1321–1332. DOI: 10.1109/TBME.2015.2512276. Epub 2015 Dec 24.
24. Parvez, M. Z.; Paul, M. Epileptic Seizure Prediction by Exploiting Spatiotemporal Relationship of EEG Signals Using Phase Correlation. *IEEE Trans. Neural Syst. Rehabil. Eng.* **2016**, *24* (1), 158–168. DOI: 10.1109/TNSRE.2015.2458982.
25. Zhang, H.; Su, J.; Wang, Q.; Liu, Y.; Good, L.; Pascual, J. Predicting Seizure by Modeling Synaptic Plasticity Based on EEG Signals—A Case Study of Inherited Epilepsy. *Commun. Nonlinear Sci. Numer. Simul.* **2017**. DOI: 10.1016/j.cnsns. 2017.08.020.
26. Park, Y.; Luo, L.; Parhi, K. K.; Netoff, T. Seizure Prediction with Spectral Power of EEG Using Cost-Sensitive Support Vector Machines. *Epilepsia* **2011**, *52* (10), 1761–1770. DOI: 10.1111/j.1528-1167.2011.03138.x.Epub 2011 Jun 21.
27. Gadhoumi, K.; Lina, J. M.; Gotman, J. Seizure Prediction in Patients with Mesial Temporal Lobe Epilepsy Using EEG Measures of State Similarity. *Clin. Neurophysiol.* **2013**, *124* (9), 1745–1754. DOI: 10.1016/j.clinph.2013.04.006. Epub 2013 May 3.
28. van der Burgh, H. K.; Schmidt, R.; Westeneng, H. J.; de Reus, M. A.; van den Berg, L. H.; van den Heuvel, M. P. Deep Learning Predictions of Survival Based on MRI in Amyotrophic Lateral Sclerosis. *Neuroimage Clin.* **2016**, *13*, 361–369. DOI: 10.1016/j.nicl.2016.10.008 (new folder 6, 1st one).

29. Breda, W.; Bremer, V.; Becker, D.; Hoogendoorn, M.; Funk, B.; Ruwaard, J.; Riper, H. Predicting Therapy Success for Treatment as Usual and Blended Treatment in the Domain of Depression. *Internet Interv.* **2018**, *12*, 100–104. New folder 2, 2nd one.
30. Schultz, J.; Becker, B.; Preckel, K.; Seifert, M.; Mielacher, C.; Conrad, R.; Kleiman, A.; Maier, W.; Kendrick, K. M.; Hurlemann, R. Improving Therapy Outcome Prediction in Major Depression Using Multimodal Functional Neuroimaging: A Pilot Study. *Pers. Med. Psychiatry* **2018**, *11–12*, 7–15.
31. Fan, F.-Y.; Li, Y.-J.; Qiu, Y.-H.; Zhu, Y.-S. Use of ANN and Complexity Measures in Cognitive EEG Discrimination. In *2005 IEEE Engineering in Medicine and Biology 27th Annual Conference*, Shanghai, 2005; pp 4638–4641. DOI: 10.1109/IEMBS.2005.1615504.
32. Li, Y.-J.; Fan, F.-Y. Classification of Schizophrenia and Depression by EEG with ANNs*. In *2005 IEEE Engineering in Medicine and Biology 27th Annual Conference*, Shanghai, 2005; pp 2679–2682. DOI: 10.1109/IEMBS.2005.1617022.
33. Acharya, U. R.; Oh, S. L.; Hagiwara, Y.; Tan, J. H.; Adeli, H.; Subha, D. P. Automated EEG-Based Screening of Depression Using Deep Convolutional Neural Network. *Comput. Methods Programs Biomed.* **2018**. DOI: 10.1016/j.cmpb.2018.04.012.
34. Kwon, O.-Y.; Park, S.-P. Depression and Anxiety in People with Epilepsy. *J. Clin. Neurol.* **2014**, *10* (3), 175–188. DOI: 10.3988/jcn.2014.10.3.175.
35. Acharya, U. R.; Hagiwara, Y.; Adeli, H. Automated Seizure Prediction. *Epilepsy Behav.* **2018**, *88*, 251–261. DOI: 10.1016/j.yebeh.2018.09.030. Epub 2018 Oct 11.
36. Mirowski, P.; Madhavan, D.; Le Cun, Y.; Kuznieck, R. Classification of Patterns of EEG Synchronization for Seizure Prediction. *Clin. Neurophysiol.* **2009**, *120* (11), 1927–1940.
37. Faust, O.; Acharya, U. R.; Adeli, H.; Adeli, A.; Wavelet-Based EEG Processing for Computer-Aided Seizure Detection and Epilepsy Diagnosis. *SEIZURE: Eur. J. Epilepsy* **2015**. http://dx.doi.org/10.1016/j.seizure.2015.01.012.
38. Cho, D.; Min, B.; Kim, J.; Lee, B. EEG-Based Prediction of Epileptic Seizures Using Phase Synchronization Elicited from Noise-Assisted Multivariate Empirical Mode Decomposition. *IEEE Trans. Neural Syst. Rehabil. Eng.* **2017**, *25* (8), 1309–1318. DOI: 10.1109/TNSRE.2016.2618937.
39. Chu, H.; Chung, C. K.; Jeon, W.; Cho, K.-H. Predicting Epileptic Seizures from Scalp EEG Based on Attractor State Analysis. *Comput. Methods Programs Biomed.* **2017**, *143*, 75–87.
40. Jauhar, S.; Krishnadas, R.; Nour, M. M.; Cunningham-Owens D.; Johnstone, E. C.; Lawrie, S. M. Is There a Symptomatic Distinction Between the Affective Psychoses and Schizophrenia? A Machine Learning Approach. *Schizophr. Res.* **2018**, *202*, 241–247. DOI: 10.1016/j.schres.2018.06.070.
41. Dipnall, J. F.; Pasco, J. A.; Berk, M.; Williams, L. J.; Dodd, S.; Jacka, F. N.; Meyer, D. Why So GLUMM? Detecting Depression Clusters Through Graphing Lifestyle-Environs Using Machine-Learning Methods (GLUMM). *Eur. Psychiatry* **2017**, *39*, 40–50. DOI: 10.1016/j.eurpsy.2016.06.003.
42. Librenza-Garcia, D.; Kotzian, B. J.; Yang, J.; Mwangi, B.; Cao, B.; Lima, P.; Nunes, L.; Bermudez, M. B.; Boeira, M. V.; Kapczinski, F.; Passos, I. C. The Impact of Machine Learning Techniques in the Study of Bipolar Disorder: A Systematic Review. *Neurosci. Biobehav. Rev.*. http://dx.doi.org/10.1016/j.neubiorev.2017.07.004.

43. Hooda, M.; Saxena, R.; Madhulika, A.; Yadav, B. A Study and Comparison of Prediction Algorithms for Depression Detection among Millennials: A Machine Learning Approach. **2017**, 779–783. DOI: 10.1109/CTCEEC.2017.8455078.
44. Khanna, A. K.; Overdyk, F. J.; Greening, C.; Di Stefano, P.; Buhre, W. F. Respiratory Depression in Low Acuity Hospital Settings-Seeking Answers from the PRODIGY Trial. *J. Crit. Care* **2018**, *47*, 80–87. DOI: 10.1016/j.jcrc.2018.06.014.
45. Gifford, G.; Crossley, N.; Fusar-Poli, P.; Schnack, H. G.; Kahn, R. S.; Koutsouleris, N.; Cannon, T. D.; McGuire, P. Using Neuroimaging to Help Predict the Onset of Psychosis. *NeuroImage* **2016**. DOI: 10.1016/j.neuroimage.2016.03.075.
46. Karim, H. T.; Wang, M.; Andreescu, C.; Tudorascu, D.; Butters, M. A.; Karp, J. F.; Reynolds C. F., 3rd; Aizenstein, H. J. Acute Trajectories of Neural Activation Predict Remission to Pharmacotherapy in Late-Life Depression. *Neuroimage Clin.* **2018**, *19*, 831–839. DOI: 10.1016/j.nicl.2018.06.006.
47. Kim, Y.-K.; Na, K.-S. Application of Machine Learning Classification for Structural Brain MRI in Mood Disorders: Critical Review from a Clinical Perspective.. *Pnp* **2017**. DOI: 10.1016/j.pnpbp.2017.06.024.
48. Sato, J. R.; Moll, J.; Green, S.; Deakin, J. F.; Thomaz, C. E.; Zahn, R. Machine Learning Algorithm Accurately Detects fMRI Signature of Vulnerability to Major Depression. *Psychiatry Res.* **2015**, *233* (2), 289–291. DOI: 10.1016/j.pscychresns.2015.07.001.
49. Patel, M. J.; Khalaf, A.; Aizenstein, H. J. Studying Depression Using Imaging and Machine Learning Methods. *Neuroimage Clin.* **2016**, *10*, 115–123.
50. Dillon, D. G.; Pizzagalli, D. A. Mechanisms of Memory Disruption in Depression. *Trends Neurosci.* **2018**, *41* (3). 137–149. DOI: 10.1016/j.tins.2017.12.006.
51. Fritz, H. B.; Vollmayr, A. S. Mechanisms of Depression: The Role of Neurogenesis. *Drug Discov. Today: Disease Mech.* **2004**, *1* (4), 407–411.
52. Alghwiri, A. A.; Khalil, H.; Al-Sharman, A.; El-Salem, K. Depression is a Predictor for Balance in People with Multiple Sclerosis. *Mult. Scler. Relat. Disord.* 2018. DOI: 10.1016/j.msard.2018.05.013.
53. Bao Y, P.; Han, Y.; Ma, J.; Wang, R. J.; Shi, L.; Wang, T. Y.; He, J.; Yue, J. L.; Shi, J.; Tang, X. D.; Lu, L. Cooccurrence and Bidirectional Prediction of Sleep Disturbances and Depression in Older Adults: Meta-Analysis and Systematic Review. *Neurosci. Biobehav. Rev.* **2017**, *75*, 257–273. DOI: 10.1016/j.neubiorev.2017.01.032.
54. Subhani, A. R.; Mumtaz, W.; Saad, M. N. B. M.; Kamel, N.; Malik, A. S. Machine Learning Framework for the Detection of Mental Stress at Multiple Levels. *IEEE Access* **2017**, *5*, 13545–13556. DOI: 10.1109/ACCESS.2017.2723622.
55. Casanova, R.; Barnard, R.; Gaussoin, S.; Saldana, S.; Hayden, K.; Manson, J. E.; Wallace, R.; Rapp, S. R.; Resnick, S. M.; Espeland, M. A.; Chen, J.-C. WHIMS-MRI Study Group and the Alzheimer's Disease Neuroimaging Initiative, Using High-Dimensional Machine Learning Methods to Estimate an Anatomical Risk Factor for Alzheimer's Disease across Imaging Databases. *NeuroImage* 2018. DOI: 10.1016/j.neuroimage.2018.08.040.
56. DeVille, D. C.; Kerr, K. L.; Avery, J. A.; Burrows, K.; Bodurka, J.; Feinstein, J.; Khalsa, S. S.; Paulus, M. P.; Simmons, W. K. The Neural Bases of Interoceptive Encoding and Recall in Healthy and Depressed Adults. *Biol. Psychiatry: Cogn. Neurosci. Neuroimaging* 2018. DOI: 10.1016/j.bpsc.2018.03.010.

57. Dey, S.; Newell, B. R.; Moulds, M. L. The Relative Effects of Abstract Versus Concrete Thinking on Decision-Making in Depression. *Behav. Res. Ther.* 2018. DOI: 10.1016/j.brat.2018.08.004.
58. Palmwood, E.; Krompinger, J. W.; Simons, R. F. Electrophysiological Indicators of Inhibitory Control Deficits in Depression. *Biol. Psychol.* https://doi.org/10.1016/j.biopsycho.2017.10.001.
59. Patel, M. J.; Khalaf, A.; Aizenstein, H. J. Studying Depression Using Imaging and Machine Learning Methods. *Neuroimage Clin.* **2016**, *10*, 115–123. DOI: https://doi.org/10.1016/j.nicl.2015.11.003.
60. Sclocco, R.; Beissner, F.; Bianciardi, M.; Polimeni, J. R.; Napadow, V. Challenges and Opportunities for Brainstem Neuroimaging with Ultrahigh Field MRI. *NeuroImage*. http://dx.doi.org/10.1016/j.neuroimage.2017.02.052.
61. Lotfaliany, M.; Bowe, S. J.; Kowal, P.; Orellana, L.; Berk, M.; Mohebbi, M. Depression and Chronic Diseases: Co-Occurrence and Communality of Risk Factors. *J. Affect. Disord.* **2018**. DOI: https://doi.org/10.1016/j.jad.2018.08.011.
62. Starlab—Living Science. [Online]. http://starlab.es/products/biosemi.
63. Allen, J.; Iacono, W.; Pepue, R.; Arbisi, P. Regional Electroencephalographic Asymmetries in Bipolar Seasonal Affective Disorder Before and After Exposure to Bright Light. *Biol. Psychiatry* **1993**, *33*, 642646.
64. Leuchter, A. F.; Cook, I. A.; Hamilton, S. P.; et al. Biomarkers to Predict Antidepressant Response. *Curr. Psychiatry Rep.* **2010**, *12* (6), 553–562.
65. Arnone, D.; Cavanagh, J.; Gerber, D.; Lawrie, S. M.; Ebmeier, K. P.; McIntosh, A. M. Magnetic Resonance Imaging Studies in Bipolar Disorder and Schizophrenia: Meta-Analysis. *Br. J. Psychiatry.* **2009**, *195* (3), 194–201.
66. Arnone, D.; McIntosh, A. M.; Ebmeier, K. P.; Munafò, M. R.; Anderson, I. M. Magnetic Resonance Imaging Studies in Unipolar Depression: Systematic Review and Meta-Regression Analyses. *Eur. Neuropsychopharmacol.* **2012**, *22* (1), 1–16.
67. Kupfer, D. J.; Frank, E.; Phillips, M. L. Major Depressive Disorder: New Clinical, Neurobiological, Andtreatment Perspectives. *Lancet* **2012**, *379*, 1045–1055.
68. Costafreda, S. G.; Chu, C.; Ashburner, J.; Fu., C. H. Prognostic and Diagnostic Potential of the Structural Neuroanatomy of Depression. *PLoS ONE* **2009**, *4* (7), e6353.
69. Agosta, F.; Pagami, E.; Petrolini, M.; Caputo, D.; Perini, M.; Prelle, A.; Salvi, F.; Filippi, M. Assessment of White Matter Tract Damage in Patients with Amyotrophic Lateral Sclerosis: A Diffusion Tensor MR Imaging Tractography Study. *AJNR Am. J. Neuroradiol.* **2010**, *31*, 1457–1561. https://dx.DOI.org/10.3174/ajnr.A2105.
70. Hoogendoom, F.; Klein, M.; Treur, M. C. Design and Analysis of an Ambient Intelligent System Supporting Depression Therapy. In *Health INF*, 2009, pp 142–148.
71. Hurley, K. D.; Van Ryzin, M. J.; Lambert, M.; Stevens, A. L. Examining Change in Therapeutic Alliance to Predict Youth Mental Health Outcomes. *J. Emotional Behav. Disord.* **2015**, *23* (2), 90–100. https://doi.org/10.1177/1063426614541700.
72. Garg, A. X.; Adhikari, N. K. J.; McDonald, H.; et al. Effects of Computerized Clinical Decision Support Systems on Practitioner Performance and Patient Outcomes: A Systematic Review. *JAMA.* **2005**, *293* (10), 1223–1238. DOI: 10.1001/jama.293.10.1223.
73. Collins, P. Y.; Patel, V.; Joestl, S. S.; March, D.; Insel, T. R.; Daar, A. S.; et al. Grand Challenges in Global Mental Health. *Nature* **2011**, *475*, 27–30. https://doi.org/10.1038/475027a.

74. Walter, M.; Lord, A. How Can We Predict Treatment Outcome for Depression? *EBioMed* **2015**, *2*, 9–10. https://doi.org/10.1016/j.ebiom.2014.12.008.
75. McGrath, C. L.; Kelley, M. E.; Holtzheimer, P. E.; Dunlop, B. W.; Craighead, W. E.; Franco, A. R.; et al. Toward a Neuroimaging Treatment Selection Biomarker for Major Depressive Disorder. *JAMA Psychiatry* **2013**, *70*, 821–829. https://doi.org/10.1001/jamapsychiatry.2013.143.
76. Hahn, T.; Nierenberg, A. A.; Whitfield-Gabrieli, S. Predictive Analytics in Mental Health: Applications, Guidelines, Challenges and Perspectives. *Mol. Psychiatry* **2016**, *22*, 37–43. https://doi.org/10.1038/mp.2016.201.
77. Papadourakis, G.; Vourkas, M.; Micheloyannis, S.; Jervis, B. W. Use of Artificaial Neural Networks for Clinical Diagnosis. *Math. Comput. Simul.* **1996**, *40*, 623–635.
78. Chen, X. S.; Wang, J. J.; Lou, F. Y. A Comparative Study of Positive and Negative Schizophrenics Using BEAM. *Acta Universitatis Medicinalis Secondae Shanghai* **2000**, *20*, 547–549.
79. Jun, G.; Smitha, K. G. EEG Based Stress Level Identification. In *Proceedings of the IEEE International Conference on System, Management and Cybernatics (SMC)*, Oct. 2016; pp 3270–3274.
80. Alonso, J. F.; Romero, S.; Ballester, M. R.; Antonijoan, R. M.; Mañanas, M. A. Stress Assessment Based on EEG Univariate Features and Functional Connectivity Measures. *Physiol. Meas.* **2015**, *36*(7), 1351.
81. Duman, R. S. Neurobiology of Stress, Depression, and Rapid Acting Antidepressants: Remodeling Synaptic Connections. *Depress. Anxiety* **2014**, *31* (4), 291–296.
82. Varatharajah, Y.; Iyer, R. K.; Berry, B. M.; Worrell, G. A.; Brinkmann, B. H. Seizure Forecasting and the Preictal State in Canine Epilepsy. *Int. J. Neural. Syst.* **2017**, *27*, 1650046 [12pp].
83. Aarabi, A.; He, B. A Rule-Based Seizure Prediction Method for Focal Neocortical Epilepsy. *Clin. Neurophysiol.* **2012**, *123*, 1111–1122.
84. Li, S.; Zhou, W.; Yuan, Q.; Liu, Y. Seizure Prediction Using Spike Rate of Intracranial EEG. *IEEE Trans. Neural Syst. Rehabil. Eng.* **2013**, *21*, 880–886.
85. Zandi, A. S.; Tafreshi, R.; Javidan, M.; Dumont, G. Predicting Epileptic Seizures in Scalp EEG Based on a Variational Bayesian Gaussian Mixture Model of Zero-Crossing Intervals. *IEEE Trans. Biomed. Eng.* **2013**, *60*, 1401–1413.
86. Zheng, Y.; Wang, G.; Li, K.; Bao, G.; Wang, J. Epileptic Seizure Prediction Using Phase Synchronization Based on Bivariate Empirical Mode Decomposition. *Clin. Neurophysiol.* **2014**, *125*, 1104–1411.
87. Teixeira, C. A.; Direito, B.; Bandarabadi, M.; van Quyen, M. I.; Valderrama, M.; Schelter, B.; et al. Epileptic Seizure Predictors Based on Computational Intelligence Techniques: A Comparative Study with 278 Patients. *Comput. Methods Programs Biomed.* **2014**, *114*, 324–336.
88. Behnam, M.; Pourghassem, H. Real-Time Seizure Prediction Using RLS Filtering and Inter Polated Histogram Feature Based on Hybrid Optimization Algorithm of Bayesian Classifier and Hunting Search. *Comput. Methods Programs Biomed.* **2016**, *132*, 115–136.
89. Sharif, B.; Jafari, A. H. Prediction of Epileptic Seizures from EEG Using Analysis of Ictal Rules on Poincare Plane. *Comput. Methods Programs Biomed.* **2017**, *145*, 11–22.

90. Günay, M.; Ensari, T. EEG Signal Analysis of Patients with Epilepsy Disorder Using Machine Learning Techniques. In *2018 Electric Electronics, Computer Science, Biomedical Engineerings' Meeting (EBBT)*, Istanbul, 2018; pp 1–4. DOI: 10.1109/EBBT.2018.8391420.
91. Kumar, P. N.; Kareemullah, H. EEG Signal with Feature Extraction Using SVM and ICA Classifiers. In *International Conference on Information Communication and Embedded Systems (ICICES2014)*, Chennai, 2014; pp 1–7. DOI: 10.1109/ICICES.2014.7034090.
92. Liu, A.; et al. Machine Learning Aided Prediction of Family History of Depression. In *2017 New York Scientific Data Summit (NYSDS)*, New York, NY, 2017; pp 1–4. DOI: 10.1109/NYSDS.2017.8085046.
93. Lisa, A. U.; Lauren, M. W.; Battlea, C. L.; Abrantesa, A. M.; Mille, I. W. Treatment Credibility, Expectancy, and Preference: Prediction of Treatment Engagement and Outcome in a Randomized Clinical Trial of Hatha Yoga vs. Health Education as Adjunct Treatments for Depression. *J. Affect. Disord.* **2018**, *238*, 111–117.
94. Mantri, S.; Patil, D.; Agrawal, P.; Wadhai, V. Non Invasive EEG Signal Processing Framework for Real Time Depression Analysis. In *2015 SAI Intelligent Systems Conference (IntelliSys)*, London, 2015; pp 518–521. DOI: 10.1109/IntelliSys.2015.7361188.
95. Prendergast, M. *Understanding Depression*; Penguin: Australia, Mar 2006.
96. Mathers, Q.; Boerma, T.; Fat, D. M. *The Global Burden of Disease: 2004 Update*; Switzerland Tech. Rep., 2004.
97. Bhattacharjee, S.; Ghatak, S.; Dutta, S.; Chatterjee, B.; Gupta, M. A Survey on Comparison Analysis Between EEG Signal and MRI for Brain Stroke Detection. *Proc. IEMIS* **2018**, *3*. DOI: 10.1007/978-981-13-1501-5_32.
98. http://sapienlabs.org/500000-human-neuroscience-papers/.
99. Balakrishnan, A.; Patapati, S. Automation of Traumatic Brain Injury Diagnosis Through an IoT-Based Embedded Systems Framework. In *2017 IEEE 8th Annual Ubiquitous Computing, Electronics and Mobile Communication Conference (UEMCON)*, 2017. DOI: 10.1109/uemcon.2017.8249087.
100. Yong, P. K.; Ho, E. T. W. Streaming Brain and Physiological Signal Acquisition System for IoT Neuroscience Application. In *2016 IEEE EMBS Conference on Biomedical Engineering and Sciences (IECBES)*, 2016. DOI: 10.1109/iecbes.2016.7843551.
101. Zhang, X.; Yao, L.; Zhang, S.; Kanhere, S.; Sheng, M.; Liu, Y. Internet of Things Meets Brain-Computer Interface: A Unified Deep Learning Framework for Enabling Human-Thing Cognitive Interactivity. *IEEE IoT J.* **2018**, *1*. DOI: 10.1109/jiot.2018.2877786.
102. Mehta, R. K.; Parasuraman, R. Neuroergonomics: A Review of Applications to Physical and Cognitive Work. *Front Hum. Neurosci.* **2013**, *7*, 889.
103. Parasuraman, R.; Wilson, G. F. Putting the Brain to Work: Neuroergonomics Past, Present, and Future. *Hum. Factors: J. Hum. Factors Ergon. Soc.* **2008**, *50*, 468–474.
104. Olokodana, I. L.; Mohanty, S. P.; Kougianos, E.; Manzo, M. Towards Photonic Sensor Based Brain-Computer Interface (BCI). In *2018 IEEE International Smart Cities Conference (ISC2)*, 2018. DOI: 10.1109/isc2.2018.8656923.
105. Cheng, M.; Gao, X.; Gao, S.; Xu, D. Design and Implementation of a Brain-Computer Interface with High Transfer Rates. *IEEE Trans. Biomed. Eng.* **2002**, *49* (10), 1181–1186. DOI: 10.1109/tbme.2002.803536.

106. Bhattacharyya, R.; Coffman, B. A.; Choe, J.; Phillips, M. E. Does Neurotechnology Produce a Better Brain? *Computer 50* (2), 48–58. DOI: 10.1109/mc.2017.49.
107. https://dzone.com/articles/applications-of-the-internet-of-things-in-the-medi-1.
108. https://www.justaskgemalto.com/en/what-is-neurotechnology/.
109. https://www.mwrf.com/systems/your-brain-iot.
110. https://www.ably.io/blog/why-iot-in-healthcare-matters.

CHAPTER 4

A STATE-OF-THE-ART SURVEY ON DECISION TREES IN THE CONTEXT OF BIG DATA ANALYSIS AND IoT

MONALISA JENA* and SATCHIDANANDA DEHURI

P.G. Department of I & CT, Fakir Mohan University, Balasore 756019, Odisha, India

*Corresponding author. E-mail: bmonalisa.26@gmail.com

ABSTRACT

In the last few decades, the expeditious expansion of the Internet and Internet of things (IoT) resulted in abrupt growth of data in almost every industry, business, and various fields of research. The embedded sensors, actuators, and software in IoT generate data in large volume and greater complexity. Analysis of these heterogeneous data with large volume and diverse dimensionalities is found to be challenging in extracting useful patterns from them and make it beneficial for the organization or society. Specialized tools are desired for analyzing and processing the huge chunk of data named "big data." Regression and classification are the fundamental tasks for data mining, pattern recognition, and big data analysis in the field of data science. The major sources of data analytics and classification task for big data are generated through embedded sensors in IoT. Soft computing is another area of research where the feature sets of an entity are quantified as some degree of fuzziness rather than exactness. A decision tree (DT) is a rule-based, recursive, and top-down tree structure widely adopted for classification and regression. DT-based algorithms play a vital role in data mining, soft computing, and big data analytics that deal with multiobjective constraints. A number of applications based on DTs have been developed to address the IoT and big data research problems. Comparative analysis of various applications of DT can be very helpful in building models with better accuracy and precision. In this work, we perform an extensive state-of-the-art survey on the role of DT in the context of soft computing, big data, and IoT.

4.1 INTRODUCTION

As technologies expand day by day, the potentiality of data generation and data collection is increasing at an exponential rate. Everywhere embedded sensors and Internet of things (IoT), which collect enormous amount of data every day, surround us. Likewise, data in today's life comes from various sources. Every day exabytes of data are produced through global telecommunication networks. A huge amount of data are generated from healthcare and medical industry at every instant of time. The data generated could be medical imaging record, patent record, doctor record, etc. As we know that the popularity of social media has been increasing at an exponential rate, the communications made through social users are the major source of digitized data. Data generated through electronic discussion networks such as blogs, emails, and web browsers are of more than thousands of terabytes every day. One of the potential sources of big data in the recent years is IoT. IoT is a way of connecting things and people anytime and anywhere, using any network and service with the help of the Internet and other technologies. Starting from the sensor implanted in holy cattle's bodies in smart farming to the sensor in our vehicles, petrol pumps, smart cities, traffic signals, sensors planted in the bed of the patient in hospitals, washing machines, ACs, and in shopping malls on clothes and doors, everywhere the things and people are connected through IoT. According to the predictions of pioneers in the particular field, over 50–100 billion devices are linked through the Internet by 2020. All the homogeneous/heterogeneous, structured/unstructured data with large volume and complexity called "big data" generated through IoT may contain useful and interesting patterns; however sometimes the data may have irrelevant and noisy information. Hence, a random analysis of this big data may lead to wastage of effort, time as well as money. Therefore, effective analysis of this data is very much crucial for the sake of betterment of various organizations and society.

In recent decades, data have been piled up from a countless number of sources at an exponential rate in the Internet. Extracting valuable information

A State-of-the-Art Survey on Decision Trees in the Context   101

from heterogeneous data accurately in timely manner is found to be a quite challenging task in the field of data science. A number of tools have been evolved in recent years to address the issues faced by data scientists. Decision tree (DT) is one of the most effective models that can extract information more accurately as compared to other models. However, their performance is related to the size of the dataset. The parallel version of DT can be adopted to reduce the computational time while processing enormous amount of data.

The rest of the chapter is organized as follows: Section 2 narrates data mining with respect to knowledge discovery in databases. Section 3 presents the decision tree induction approach for classification. Section 4 illustrates soft computing aspects with reference to the decision tree classifier. The traditional approach for data analysis is discussed in Section 5. The preliminary concepts, issues and technologies in big data analysis and IoT has been discussed in Sections 6 and 7 respectively. The application of decision tree concerning big data and IoT is described in Section 8, and Section 9 concludes the chapter.

4.2 DATA MINING

Data mining is the process of wrenching out useful and interesting data patterns from the unprocessed raw datasets.[1] Until and unless a piece of rock is mined, it cannot be ascertained whether some precious material is hidden inside it or it is simply a piece of rock/sand. Data mining is one of the most important phases in the process of knowledge discovery in databases (KDD). It can be defined as the process of exploring hidden, valuable pattern from data. The pattern discovered is desired to be unambiguous, novel, and comprehensive in nature.[2,3] The various steps followed in KDD process are presented as follows[3]:

1. Identifying the application domain: There should be a proper knowledge regarding the domain of the datasets to be selected and objectives of the application.
2. Data cleaning and integration: In real world, data sources are many a time incomplete, inconsistent, and imprecise, maybe due to some inadequacy in the implementation or error in the operations. Data cleaning involves noise removal and handling of missing data. Data from heterogeneous, multiple data sources are integrated to extract best features from them.

3. Data selection: The database consists of several kinds of data, of which not all are relevant for the analysis task. Hence, an appropriate selection method needs to be chosen for extracting the valuable data required for the analysis.
4. Transformation and reduction of data: As the raw data contains much noisy information, the data need to be transformed into an appropriate form by applying various aggregation techniques after the selection. Sometimes it is necessary to have dimension reduction in order to eradicate the noisy data. Depending on the objectives of the task, useful features are obtained to represent the data, and in case of large datasets, data reduction is performed using efficient dimensionality reduction techniques.
5. Choosing the data mining functions and algorithms: It involves determining the appropriate functions and algorithms to be used for finding patterns in the data. Different data mining algorithms have different purposes. Different methods such as classification, regression, clustering, image segmentation/classification, link analysis, functional dependencies, and rule extraction are used based on the requirements, and hence, appropriate models are constructed accordingly.
6. Data mining: It includes extraction of data patterns of interest in a specific representational form by applying intelligent methods.
7. Pattern evaluation: After extracting the patterns, it is necessary to analyze and evaluate them to recognize the truly interesting patterns.
8. Knowledge representation: The discovered patterns are interpreted and possible visualizations are being done to represent the mined knowledge to users. This knowledge is incorporated into the performance system.

The whole KDD process is depicted in Figure 4.1.

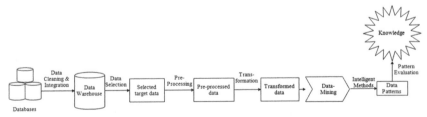

FIGURE 4.1 Data mining as a step in KDD.[11]

4.2.1 CLASSIFICATION IN DATA MINING

Several techniques such as classification, clustering, regression, characterization, discrimination, and many more exist in data mining. In this chapter, our main focus is on classification through rule-based model such as DT. Classification is a process of partitioning the objects into specific labels, which depends on the set of features or characteristics they have. It consists of two phases. In the first phase, the model is being trained on a set of objects (training data). It is known as learning phase. After the model passes through sufficient data, it is being tested by another set of objects (testing data) for performance evaluation. The major objective of the classifier model is to extract the classification rules from the training data and apply those rules on testing data to get the desired result. Classification rules are nothing but prediction rules composed of a list of conditional[6-8] statements that may have IF-ELSE statements. The IF construct may have the set of constraints independent of the attributed value and the ELSE construct has the result that depends on the set of statements discovered at the IF part. Each pair of antecedent and consequent is known as a rule. The general form of RULE: Antecedent: IF ($cond_1$ AND $cond_2$ AND ...AND $cond_n$) → Consequent: THEN (the predicted class label). In this rule, each constraint mentioned in the IF part can be represented as x opr t. Here x is an attribute and t denotes a value against which the attribute is compared, and opr is a comparison operator of form $opr \in \{=, \neq, >, <, \leq, \geq\}$.

The second step is called the classification step, in which the performance of the classification rules is measured using test data, and if it is up to the mark, the rules are applied on unknown data tuples to predict their class labels. Several classifiers such as Bayesian classifier and *k*-nearest neighbor classifier exist in the field of data mining, of which our area of interest is DT classifier. It is an efficient and easy-to-understand classifier, the performance of which is comparable with many promising classifiers.

4.3 DECISION TREE

A DT is one of the most effective rule-based machine-learning approaches that can be represented through tree data structure. The internal nodes containing conditions applied on attributes are called decision nodes,[9] branches denote outcomes of the condition, and leaf nodes hold class labels in the classifier. The topmost node is the root or parent of the tree.

Figure 4.2 represents a sample DT[10] for the concept "raining," that is, based on the conditions imposed on, the DT will predict whether it will rain or not. In the figure, the internal nodes are represented in the form of ovals and class labels in the form of rectangles. The features are temperature (temp), wind, and pressure and the two class labels are *rain* and *no rain*. The class prediction for a tuple can be represented by drawing a path from the root node to the child node where at each node a set of constraints has been defined. For example, for the tuple (temp > 75 °F, wind > 2.5 mph, and pressure > 25 Hg), the class label is "rain." Like this, various rules are extracted from the DT, and using those rules, the class label of unseen sample is predicted. In the diagram, temp is taken as the root node. The selection of root node is not done haphazardly. Using several attribute selection measures, such as entropy, gain ratio, and Gini index, and the splitting criterion used by them, splitting attribute is selected for a particular node.

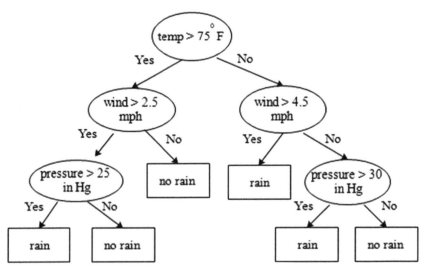

FIGURE 4.2 A decision tree example.[46]

4.3.1 DT INDUCTION

The training phase of the DT is known as DT induction. In this phase, the model tries to extract the set of rules from the training objects that are associated with the set of features along with the class labels. While

A State-of-the-Art Survey on Decision Trees in the Context 105

inducing a DT, one important factor to be considered is splitting criterion.[11,12] The splitting criterion helps us in choosing the attribute that partitions the tuples in the dataset into individual classes by making a test at node N. Using the splitting attribute, we can determine either a possible split point or a splitting subset based on the DT induction algorithm used. The dataset is partitioned in the aim that all samples in the partitions of a dataset are linked to the same class. Such a partition is said to be pure. For an attribute t having x values $t_1, t_2, \ldots, t_x$, if it is discrete-valued, a branch labeled with each attribute values is created for the same. If it is continuous, then possible splits are of the form $t \leq c$ for one partition and $t > c$ for the other, where c is the split point. If the attribute is discrete and binary trees are to be generated only, then the splitting is of the form $t \in S_t$, where S_t is the splitting subset for t. Figure 4.3 depicts the scenario.

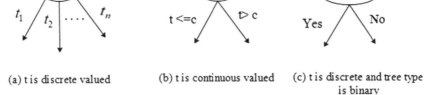

(a) t is discrete valued   (b) t is continuous valued   (c) t is discrete and tree type is binary

FIGURE 4.3   Splitting based on attributes.[11]

4.3.2 ADVANTAGES OF DT

- It divides original dataset into significant subgroups making complex relationships between predictor variables and response variables simpler.
- It is comprehensible and interpretable.
- It does not use any distributional assumptions, rather uses nonparametric approach.
- It easily handles missing values using imputation methods[13] and sometimes without using imputation.
- It also handles outliers effectively.
- It can handle the datasets of larger dimensions either by applying dimensionality reduction techniques prior to classification or by partitioning the large dataset into smaller subsets. This can be

achieved through computing each subset independently in parallel manner, and the result of each computation is then combined to get desired output.

While constructing a DT, two characteristics need to be simultaneously considered: complexity and robustness. With the increase in complexity, the reliability of predicting new data sample decreases. If it is desired to make each leaf node 100% pure, then the resultant DT will be highly complex in structure as each leaf node will consist of very few records.[14] Such a situation leads to overfitting of the DT; so, it cannot reliably predict unseen data tuples and thus might lead to lack of robustness. Hence, stopping rules need to be imposed while constructing a DT to reduce the complexity. Stopping parameters such as the minimum number of tuples at a terminal node and the minimum number of tuples before splitting must be chosen based on the goal of the analysis and the characteristics of the dataset being used. However, in some situations, the stopping rules do not perform well. An alternative approach to deal with overfitting is tree pruning.

4.3.3 TREE PRUNING

It is an effective method of handling the issue of overfitting. Pruning in DT can be performed in two ways: prepruning and postpruning. The first one involves halting the growth of the tree at an early stage by making decision at a node not to stretch it further. The leaf node may contain the class having the highest frequency among the subset of tuples or the probability distribution of the tuples present in the subset.[11] Using chi-square tests or other comparison adjustment methods, the production of less significant branches can be halted in case of *prepruning*. For example, if at a particular node, the result of chi-square test or other measures of statistical significance such as entropy and Gini index is less than a prespecified threshold, then the branches that generate from that node become insignificant. Hence, their growing should be halted. In case of *postpruning*, it deletes unwanted branches after constructing a fully grown DT in a manner that improves the accuracy of the overall classification. In this method, the nodes that provide less information are removed by producing an optimal DT, and they are replaced with a class label as the terminal node. The terminal node contains the class having highest occurrence in the replaced subtree.

For example, in the DT of Figure 4.2, the frequency of class label "rain" is more in comparison to class label "no rain." Hence, if post pruning is applied, the right subtree can be replaced with class label "rain" that becomes a leaf node. The process is depicted in Figure 4.4.

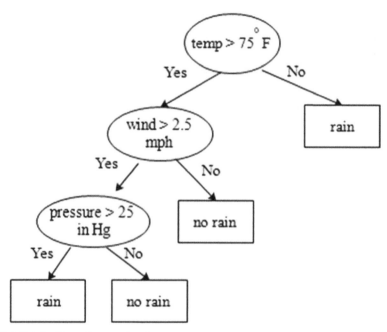

FIGURE 4.4 Tree after pruning.[46]

4.4 SOFT COMPUTING ASPECTS IN DECISION TREE CLASSIFIER

It has been observed that getting exact solution to real-world complex problems is quite a challenging task. Soft computing is an alternative model to get approximate solution for many complex problems.[15] Unlike hard computing, it allows the researchers to handle uncertainty, fuzziness, and imprecision existing in the dataset. The mechanism behind soft computing can be assumed to be derived from the human brain. The major areas that come under the umbrella of soft computing can be genetic algorithm (GA), artificial neural network (ANN), rule-based expert systems and fuzzy logic, etc. All of the soft-computing paradigms aim to quantify the degree of uncertainty or tolerance level in imprecision in order to get the solution for the complicated problems.

DT is one of the most effective ways for handling classification and regression problems where at each step, a number of decisions based on certain constraints need to be taken. The number as well as the order of the decisions to be taken at each step can be obtained through soft-computing paradigms as mentioned previously. Some of the soft-computing paradigms are discussed later.

4.4.1 GENETIC ALGORITHM (GA)

GAs are proved effective for implementing DT algorithms. This evolutionary algorithm is derived from the nature-inspired Darwin's genetic evolution. The intuition behind this approach is that the best optimal solution for a problem can be obtained by combining the best features of already known solutions. The degree of suitability of a solution is measured by the fitness function that is the basic objective function for the problem. The following steps illustrate the major steps followed in GA:

> Step 1: Choose the appropriate encoding scheme that is suitable for solving the problem. It is usually problem specific.
>
> Step 2: Initialize the population by generating chromosomes or the solutions randomly with the help of chosen encoding scheme.
>
> Step 3: Calculate the fitness of the chromosomes based on the objective function that needs to be devised before the actual processing starts.
>
> Step 4: Choose the appropriate selection method for keeping the best individuals in the population. This is used to eradicate the infeasible solutions to the problem. The degree of convergence of the population toward optimal solution depends on the chosen selection method.
>
> Step 5: Apply the genetic operators such as mutation and crossover to generate population for the next generation.
>
> Step 6: Repeat steps 3–5 till the population converge to the optimal solution or the stopping criteria satisfied.

Most of the DT induction algorithms follow the top-down greedy approach where recursive partitioning of the dataset is carried out. However, it may lead to an overfitting problem as the size of the dataset becomes too small to select the attributes at each level. One of the solutions to this problem may be ensemble of various induction DTs in order to construct the classification model. The outcome of the classification task can be obtained by voting of result from different DTs. It may be prone to some of the limitations as if it may have high inconsistency results among the several trees, especially when comprehensiveness of the single DT matters. Evolutionary algorithm such as GA is one of the suitable alternatives to address this problem. Unlike local search, GA looks for the global search in the population space.

A case study may be considered for clear understanding of GA application in modeling the DT algorithm. Liu et al. have presented a mobile user classification problem based on the DT classifier modeled from GA. In their case study, mobile users are classified based on the services they are interested in. They are classified into four different categories such as basic service user, e-service user, plus service user, and total service user. The basic task of any DT algorithm is to generate a set of rules with single or multiobjective constraints that will lead to correct classification. DT algorithm often leads to inaccurate classification as it often fails to get optimized rules, which is a cumbersome task. An objective function can be designed based on the attributes (gain ratio, support, accuracy, simplicity, etc.) associated with the rules. This objective function can be treated as the fitness function for GA. Genetic operators such as mutation and crossover can be put in to maximize the fitness value that in turn optimizes the rules at each level of the DT. The proposed approach presented in the case study is described in Figure 4.5.

4.4.2 FUZZY APPLICATION IN MODELING DT

DT is the suitable classifier to extract the rules from the set of instances in order to predict the class labels of unseen samples. However, it fails to capture the uncertainty involved in the datasets. Fuzzy DT (FDT) is one of such extensions to address the vagueness involved in the datasets. It tries to learn the pattern from the pool of instances and presents the result through the fuzzy representation. The FDT classifier comprises the following steps:

1. Fuzzy partitioning
2. Induction of FDT
3. Fuzzy rule inference for classification

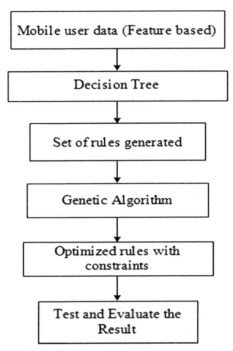

FIGURE 4.5 Case study: mobile user classification using decision tree with genetic algorithm.[47]

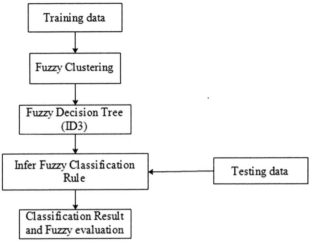

FIGURE 4.6 Architecture of FDT.[48]

Fuzzy partitioning is the first step in the classification process where input dataset is divided into partitions using standard fuzzy clustering techniques. FDT is then constructed using any DT algorithm such as ID3. The architecture of FDT[16,17] is presented in Figure 4.6. Recursive top-down partitioning and divide-and-conquer approach are adopted at this step. Fuzzy entropy measure is applied at each level to determine the high influential attribute for node splitting. The recursive node splitting is carried out until the stopping criteria are satisfied. Some[18] of the stopping criteria may be as described as follows:

- If the number of pattern processed is less than the threshold, the branch terminates and acts as a leaf node.
- If, in a path, suitable attribute does no more exist for splitting, the branch terminates.
- If the path is not converging after exceeding certain path length, the branch terminates.

A wide number of algorithms are available to model the FDT. The classification ability of these algorithms can be evaluated through various measures such as average fuzzy classification ambiguity, average fuzzy classification entropy, and fuzzy rough interactive.

4.4.3 ARTIFICIAL NEURAL NETWORK (ANN)

ANN is the classification model that functions similar to the natural brain. The basic element of the neural network is the neuron that resembles with the neuron cell present in our brain. It is nothing but a network of neuron cells that are having some activating capacity to process the signal that passes through it. It is the most popular tool in the field of data science especially when classification task is concerned. However, it is quite complex and difficult to understand the underlying processing mechanism. In order to make it more reliable and better understandable, the architecture of neural network can be mapped into DT model. ANN model may be considered as a layered architecture that consists of one input layer, one output layer, and one or more hidden layers. It has been observed that ANN works perfectly for large size datasets. However, when it is mapped with DT, the nodes available at lower level are used by very less fraction of training data. As a result, the leaf nodes tend to overfit unless sufficient large amount of data is available as compared to the depth of the tree. The DT model built to illustrate the simplification of the process carried out in neural network can be called as soft DT. In this tree, a bias value and weight are assigned at each node, further resulting in a distribution probability. The leaf node having the highest probability will be the source of output generator.

4.5 TRADITIONAL APPROACH FOR DATA ANALYSIS

Earlier data were stored in databases such as DB2, MS SQL Server, or Oracle databases, and sophisticated software were used to process the data for data analysis purpose. A user interacts with a centralized server to fetch and analyze data from the database. The interaction between user and database is shown in Figure 4.7.

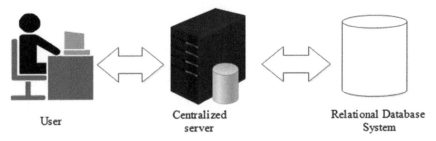

FIGURE 4.7 Interaction in traditional data processing system.[49]

4.5.1 *LIMITATION*

Traditional approach suits well for users dealing with less volume of data. While dealing with datasets of high dimensionality, it is perceived that traditional database server cannot handle them efficiently. In a traditional system, storing and retrieving volumes of data had three major issues: cost, speed, and reliability. So, to overcome this, these days big data analysis techniques are adopted by various organizations across the world.

4.6 BIG DATA ANALYSIS

In today's world, the digitalization of our daily activities has resulted in enormous amount of data that is of large volume, greater complexity, and high dimensionality. This data, called "big data," is used by many organizations to extract valuable information[19] from them for either taking financial decisions, tracking specific behaviors, tracing patient's health condition, or to detect threat attacks.[20] The processing of such data is very much difficult by the traditional database analysis techniques. Hence, powerful and effective techniques, called big data analytics (BDA), are desired by the organizations that can deal with any massive volume of heterogeneous, unstructured, structured, and semistructured data that are growing day by day expeditiously.

4.6.1 CHARACTERISTICS OF BIG DATA (FOUR V'S)

BDA can be better explained from the concept of four V's as follows:

Volume: It represents the amount or quantity of data that may range from MB (megabytes) to PB (petabytes) of data.

Velocity: It defines the rate at which data are generated and delivered to the end users.

Variety: It represents data from a different variety. In real world, data can be of structured, semistructured, or unstructured form. Data can again be of homogeneous and heterogeneous types depending on whether the data are of the same type or mixed type.

Veracity: It says data generated and used should be unambiguous, bias-free, and trustworthy.

Hence, big data can be defined as data having high volume, high velocity, and/or high variety and veracity. It requires new methods and technologies to accumulate, apprehend, and analyze and is used to magnify decision-making process, deliver proper understanding and discovery, and optimize processes.[6] Figure 4.8 depicts the four V's with examples in respective areas.

4.6.2 HOW DOES BIG DATA WORK?

With the development of modern tools and technologies, it is possible to perform different operations on larger datasets and extract valuable information from them by analyzing the behaviors of patterns in the datasets. Big data technologies make it technically and economically feasible. Big data mainly addresses the scalability and complexity issues that appear in the traditional approaches within a reasonable elapsed time. It mainly refers to the large and complex datasets that are not conventionally analyzed by traditional database systems. It needs a set of new techniques and technologies in order to extract useful information from datasets that are heterogeneous in nature. Processing of big data involves different steps that begin from collection of raw information to implementation of actionable information.

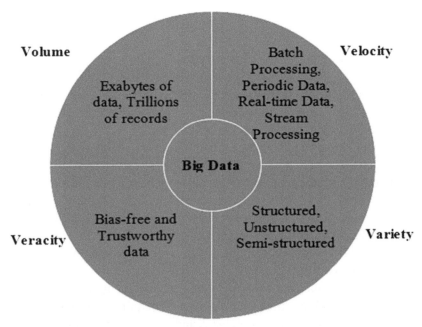

FIGURE 4.8 Four V's of big data analytics.[50]

Collection of data: Many organizations face different challenges and hurdles at the beginning while dealing with big data. Such challenges are mobile devices, logs, raw data transactions, social sites, etc. However, these challenges can be conquered by a proper big data platform, and developers are allowed to ingest the data from the different variety.

Storing: Preprocessed and postprocessed data need to be stored in a secure, durable, and scalable repository system. This is an essential step for any big data platform. Depending on the particular requirements, a user can opt for the temporary storage of data.

Processing and Analyzing: Transformation of raw data into user consumable data by various stages such as sorting, joining, and aggregation is necessary. The result datasets are stored and used for any further processing tasks.

Consuming and Visualizing: Finally, an end user gets the valuable insights from the processed datasets, and according to the requirements, the user plans for the future strategies.

4.6.3 ISSUES IN BIG DATA

Since the last few years, almost every sector is generating enormous amount of data that need big data technologies to process them in order to analyze and make business decision. Several sectors such as healthcare department, education institutes, administrative departments, national security, banking sector, and e-commerce[21,22] business are the leading organizations in the world of big data. Every financial transaction, ticket reservation in airlines, railway, and usage of social media lead to generation of huge amount of data every day. Big data research has been extended to many interdisciplinary research areas such as biochemistry, biotechnology, agriculture, pharmaceutical, computer science, electrical, astronomy, and atmospheric science. Apart from these areas, some of the very popular applications in social media[23,24] such as Twitter, Facebook, Yahoo, and many recommendation and search engines encounter big data problem frequently. The widely adopted technologies in IoT are also contributing a lot as countless sensors and actuators around us every day. From this discussion, it can be observed that big data problem has been spreading into several domains. Some of them are briefly discussed later.

4.6.3.1 BIG DATA ANALYTICS IN SOCIAL NETWORK

In the last few decades, the observation shows that more than 30,000 GB of data are generated at each minute with a great rate of acceleration. These data are generated from a variety of sources that make them heterogeneous in nature. The major sources of data are mainly from social networks. Social networks are always loaded with blog posts, text messages, audios, videos, etc. The ultimate source of data is the Internet that is almost indecipherable. Applications such as Facebook, Yahoo, Friendster, and

Twitter in social network domain not only allow the users to be connected through social relationship but also generate tens of exabytes of data from their frequent social interaction.[22] Several messenger applications such as WhatsApp, Snapchat, and Facebook Messenger allow exchange of text messages, voice as well as video calls, images, documents, other media, and user locations, which leads to deposition of large amount of complex and heterogeneous data. By analyzing this information kept in the social networks such as Twitter, Instagram, WhatsApp, and Facebook, marketing agencies predict the future strategies.

4.6.3.2 BIG DATA IN SCIENTIFIC RESEARCH

Scientific research in the fields of bioinformatics, social computing, computer science, astrology, microbiology, astrophysics, and computational theory leads to a variety of data driven applications that artificially generate vast amount of synthetic data in order to make extensive research. However, it is a quite challenging task to explore the pattern or valuable information from the raw data generated from complex scientific simulation. These research fields could be the potential candidates for big data problem. For example, astronomers can apply advanced analysis methods on the image data recorded by a sophisticated telescope, and using the result of the analysis, they can identify the pattern for the evolution of the universe. Human genome also contains huge volume of information, decoding which is a tedious and time-consuming task. It is observed that, in all these disciplines, enormous data are generated on a regular basis; hence, advanced and automated analysis techniques are highly desired. In addition to this, a centralized repository is necessary to keep the records of different research groups as a backup.

4.6.3.3 BIG DATA IN COMMERCE AND BUSINESS

Like social network and scientific research areas, commerce and business is also one of the important sources of big data. There are millions of shopping malls across the world in which millions of transactions are taking place every day leading to accumulation of huge amount of data every day. The hidden patterns in big data can be extracted by applying sophisticated machine learning techniques using which the business organizations can build accurate business models in order to improve their product recommendation strategy. This would also help them to make efficient decision strategy. The transactions carried out by the customers of multinational companies present across the world also have huge contribution in the field of big data. Business organizations learn behaviors of their consumers about their products using the information in the social media such as product perception and preferences. Nowadays, e-commerce is the more preferable source of purchase by customers. Therefore, daily lot of purchase and transactions is taking place leading to a generation of enormous amount of data, which includes customer's information details, transaction details, search details, and many more. Hence, implementation of BDA techniques into e-commerce leads to higher productivity as compared to their competitors.[25] Even though BDA tools are expensive, still they save a lot of money, helping to reduce the extra burdens of business leaders and analysts.

4.6.3.4 BIG DATA IN HEALTHCARE

The healthcare sector contributes a large portion of electronic data toward the era of big data, which is quite difficult to process in traditional tools and data management technologies. The large volume of data in healthcare department allows the doctors to identify the accurate pattern and detect the disease at an early stage. However, it may take longer time to process than expected due to its large volume of data.[26] By effectively analyzing the big data with appropriate technology, the patient can be treated easily, which ultimately leads to reduction of health complications. Sometimes healthcare fraud can be detected by mapping the sample pattern with the population[27,28] pattern in the big data. A number of patient reports such as life span of patient, the type of surgery they are choosing, complications associated with the patients, disease progress, and test report results can be analyzed to provide better and quicker services in healthcare sector.

4.6.3.5 BIG DATA IN SOCIETY ADMINISTRATION

Big data has also been a part of administrative systems in the society. The world population is increasing at a rapid rate. Different age-group people want variety of public services from their administration. For example, the children and the teenagers require better education system, young people need information about the jobs, middle-aged persons require better livelihood, and the elder persons are looking for better healthcare system in the society. Each of the groups is accumulating different variety of data in public repository that leads to high volume of big data. These data may be used by the administrator to provide better service. As the data size is increasing at the repository at an exponential rate, handling all the issues has becoming quite challenging by using traditional tools. Powerful administrators along with efficient big data technologies need to be adopted to provide the services in timely manner. With the help of effective tools and technologies for analyzing big data, the heavy budget and debt level may be reduced dramatically at the administrative level.[7]

4.7 INTERNET OF THINGS

IoT also known as Internet of everything is a way of connecting devices such as sensors, actuators, mobile phones, radio frequency identifiers (RFID), and others to the Internet through unique addressing schemes and standard communication protocols to reach common goals.[29] The concept of IoT was proposed by Kevin Ashton in 1999. The IoT is considered as one of the promising areas of future technology and is the area of interest of several industries and organizations. The idea of connecting everything over the Internet makes it the point of attraction of everybody. Figure 4.9 shows a scenario in which the devices are connected through IoT.[30-32]

To know IoT in detail, we need to discuss the key technologies that have been adopted in recent years. Some of the important technologies are briefly discussed later.

4.7.1 RADIO FREQUENCY IDENTIFICATION (RFID)

RFID is the technology that reveals the identity and captures the data with the help of RFID device or Tag, a tag reader, and radio wave.[33] Objects or people are detected automatically with the help of radio waves. The major components of RFID technology are the RFID device, tag reader with transceiver, and antenna that capture the data with radio waves. RFID is found to have better performance as compared to other bar code reader as it assigns a unique tag for each object through which it collects the information about the object by using some tag reader. The tags used in RFID system can be of two types: active and passive. Active tags are supplied with battery and can perform read/write operations, whereas there is no power supply provided to passive tag that is read-only in nature. Passive tags are smaller, lighter, and less expensive than active tags. Passive tags have unlimited life, whereas active tags have limited life because of the battery, but with the current battery technology, the life span of batteries has increased as much as 10 years. Apart from these two, semipassive tags act as an intermediary between active and passive tags where the circuit is being power supplied by drawing the power from either the battery or the tag reader. Because of its better functionality, its cost is higher than the passive tag. The chips in RFID tags contain electronic product code (EPC) number and readers identify the EPC number without any physical contact or scanning. Middleware is used to perform data filtering from the readers' data. A wide number of big data applications such as animal husbandry, postal tracking, supply chain tracking, airline baggage management software, toll collection, vehicle parking access control, monitoring of offenders, and railway rolling stock identification use RFID as their major component.

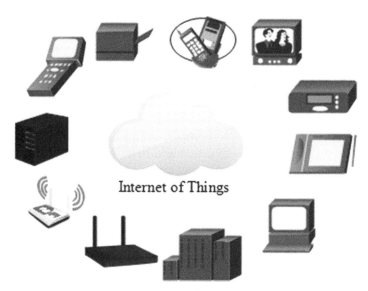

FIGURE 4.9 Devices connected through IoT.[51]

4.7.2 WIRELESS SENSOR NETWORKS (WSN)

Sensors are intelligent, smaller, and, these days, cheaper devices equipped with wireless interfaces to communicate with one another forming a network.[36] Wireless sensor network (WSN) consists of a number of autonomous devices each attached[34,35] with a variety of sensors distributed over multidimensional space used to capture the parameters of objects such as position, temperature, humidity, and motions.[37] Smart sensor nodes in WSN are usually equipped with multiple sensors, an actuator, a radio, a processing unit, and a battery to supply the power and memory for storage. Since sensors are miniature devices, they have very restricted amount of storage capacity. Unlike other computing devices, they usually have a very limited functionality in accessing location information about other nodes. They use the radio web for transferring the data to an access point or to any base station. According to the suitableness of the environment, solar panels may also be implemented as a secondary source of power supply to the nodes. Sensors can be of various types such as chemical, biological, magnetic, thermal, mechanical, and optical, and depending on the purpose of usage and nature of environment, actuators are deployed in the sensors.

WSNs are of two types: structured and unstructured. An unstructured WSN consists of a vast collection of sensor nodes. In this network, as there are so many nodes, network maintenance and failure detection are very difficult. Once the sensor node is deployed, the monitoring and reporting functions in the network are not tracked continuously. In contrast to this, sensor nodes are deployed in a predetermined manner in structured WSN. In a structured network, lesser nodes are deployed with much less management cost and network maintenance.

WSNs have applications in various fields such as in retail stores for keeping track of materials and goods, in military target tracking and surveillance system for identification and helping in intrusion detection, monitoring patient's health condition in biomedical health monitoring system, in natural disaster relief to sense and detect disasters a priori, and in earthquake-prone and volcanic-eruption areas for detection of earthquake and eruption much before it happens.

4.7.3 MIDDLEWARE

It is a software layer intervened between the application levels and technological levels. It provides interactions among heterogeneous sensors, actuators, and context aware applications without hampering privacy and security issues. It presents multiple services and provides abstraction to the applications from objects or things. IoT having a complicated and distributed architecture needs a simplified approach for the development of new applications and services. In recent years, IoT follows the service-oriented architecture (SOA) for most of the middleware. The employment of SOA approach helps in solving the large and complex applications into simpler ones. Therefore, the middleware plays a vital role in IoT application development.

4.7.4 CLOUD COMPUTING

Cloud computing is a framework providing a huge number of configurable, convenient resources such as computers, servers, networks, storage, applications, and services online on demand basis.[38] The virtually unlimited resources of cloud can overcome the technological constraints in IoT such as communication, storage, and processing. The devices connected to the Internet through IoT generate enormous amount of data hence require huge data storage and high processing speed. Cloud provides solutions to the data collection and complex data processing in IoT by enabling rapid setup and amalgamation of new things yet maintaining low costs for setup and integration. Figure 4.10 shows the three service models of cloud: software as a service (SaaS), platform as a service (PaaS), and infrastructure as a service (IaaS). In SaaS, software is used as a service. It utilizes the Internet to deliver applications. Some examples are Google Apps, Cisco WebEx, etc. Application developers manage PaaS. PaaS provides a proper framework for developers to create certain software and customized applications. Google App Engine, Apache Stratos, etc. are the examples of PaaS. IaaS provides infrastructure to those organizations that do not have proper infrastructure as per their needs. It is managed by infrastructure and network architects.

4.7.5 IoT APPLICATION SOFTWARE

IoT applications allow device-to-device and human-to-device interactions in an authentic and robust manner. The IoT applications should ensure the timely delivery and action of messages/data. IoT applications for human-to-device interactions require data visualization to provide instinctive and easy-to-understand information to the end users and they permit communion with the environment. The IoT applications should be designed with intelligence so that devices can communicate with each other, recognize the problems, resolve the problems, and track the environmental condition without any human intervention.

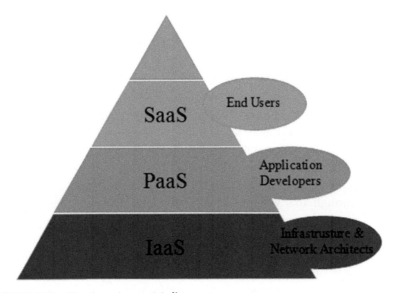

FIGURE 4.10   Cloud service models.[51]

4.8   DECISION TREE FOR BIG DATA ANALYSIS AND IoT

The electronic data are growing very fast and especially the data generated through IoT are growing at an exponential rate. Hence, applying traditional data analysis methods to this large amount of data is potentially time-consuming and the result is unsatisfactory. Accumulation of this huge amount of data called big data in computer system may engulf the memory and lead to slow processing. Finding interesting patterns in these huge amounts of data is a tedious task. One method is to divide the large dataset into subsets and distribute the data and computations among several processors and memories.[39] The parallel processing is done with the help of DT. The strategy is to divide the original big dataset into n partitions and construct DTs learning from the class labeled tuples of each partition. A DT is grown independently on each of n processors and after that, they must be combined using some strategies. Some of the researchers used metalearning approach in which the outputs of individual tree classifiers are combined based on some metarules.[40] Therefore, the goal is to combine the independent trees into a single DT. Rules are extricated from each of the DT at n nodes and then the rules are integrated into a single rule set. At a time, only two rule sets are merged. Then using single rule set, the unknown data tuples are classified. While deploying the process of partitioning and merging, it happens that the size of the independent trees becomes very large as they are part of the big dataset. Similarly, the length of the rules also increases rapidly leading to the curse of dimensionality problem.[41] To reduce the size of the tree, pruning must be applied. Rules can be extracted from pruned as well as unpruned trees.

However, some complications are involved in the process. Some rules conflict each other if the classes in the overlapping regions are unlike. So, in that case, combining them is not feasible. Therefore, the conflicting rules must be resolved before combining them. There may be some rules having same conditions but different conditional test results. These rules can be combined to single rule sets. Several procedures are applied to solve conflicts.[39,42,] One of them is to first find all the rule pairs having equal "if" conditions, and the attributes used in the pairs are same but the attribute values taken in the condition are different. For example, if attribute values are continuous for the attribute "x," then the test condition[43-45] is of the form $x > 2.5$ in one rule, and in other rule, the condition is of the form $x > 3.2$. If the test condition is of $>$ form, then the lesser of the two values is used. In the previous example, $x > 2.5$ is considered as the combined rule of the set. If the condition is of $\leq$ form, then the greater of the two attributes' values is considered for the combined rule. For example, if two conditions are $x \leq 9$ and $x \leq 6$, then $x \leq 9$ is used in the combined rule. The next step is to recognize all the pairs of rules those have approximately all conditions same and have different class labels. These are said to be conflicting rules. For example, consider the following two rules:

Rule 1— $x > 0.5$ and $y > 0.8$: class 1 and
Rule 2— $x > 0.5$ and $z \leq 0.7$: class 2. Where x, y, and z are attributes of the dataset.

The previous two rules are having the same first condition but they differ in the second. These are conflicting rules. The rules can be made stronger by adding some negations to the conditions, which mismatch. In the previous case, negation of $y > 0.8$ will be $y \leq 0.8$. It will be added to rule 2. Similarly $z > 0.7$ will be added to rule 1. Hence, the modified rules can be written as:

MRule 1— $x > 0.5$ and $y > 0.8$ and $z > 0.7$: class 1 and
MRule 2— $x > 0.5$ and $z \leq 0.7$ and $y \leq 0.8$: class 2.

If all the conflicting examples, which match the previous conditions, belong to the same class, then the rule is taken as final. If they belong to mixed classes, then a new condition is found and imposed that helps in dividing the dataset into pure partitions. Now the new rule can be written as:

MRule 11— $x > 0.5$ and $y > 0.8$ and cond.: class 1 and
MRule 12— $x > 0.5$ and $y > 0.8$ and cond. class 2.

Next step is to eliminate redundancies, if any in the conditions. For example, if there is a rule $y > 0.3$ and $z < 0.8$ and $y > 0.5$: class 2, then the condition $y > 0.3$ is redundant as it is included in the last condition. So it is eliminated. Then Step 2 is repeated to check if there are any conflicting rules.

If not, Step 1 is repeated and then the two rule sets are merged and redundancies raised, if any, during the process of elimination of conflicts are removed.

4.9 CONCLUSION

DT classifier is one of the most popular and simplified models considered in the field of data science. It has been observed that DT performs well for both classification and regression tasks of data mining. However, the performance of the model is limited with the size of the dataset. Although it is simple to understand the underlying mechanism, its computational complexity is high for large-size datasets. The major objective of DT is to explore the set of rules along with their constraints from the database, which can be arranged into a treelike structure for better representation. It has been widely adopted in a number of applications in IoT and big data where enormous data has been piled up every day. In this chapter, we have presented various issues and applications of DT in the field of IoT, big data, and soft computing. Unlike hard computing, DT can be the potential solution for many complex problems in the field of soft computing where approximate solution with better accuracy is desired instead of exact solution with poor accuracy. Different issues for DT in the field of soft computing paradigms such as GA, ANN, and fuzzy logic have also been presented in this chapter.

KEYWORDS

- data mining
- big data analysis
- decision tree
- IoT
- soft computing

REFERENCES

1. Chen, M. S.; Han, J.; Yu, P. S. Data Mining: An Overview from a Database Perspective. *IEEE Trans. Knowl. Data Eng.* **1996,** *8* (6), 866–883.
2. Liao, S. H.; Chu, P. H.; Hsiao, P. Y. Data Mining Techniques and Applications—A Decade Review from 2000 to 2011. *Expert Syst. Appl.* **2012,** *39* (12), 11303–11311.
3. Mitra, S.; Pal, S. K.; Mitra, P. Data Mining in Soft Computing Framework: A Survey. *IEEE Trans. Neural Netw.* **2002,** *13* (1), 3–14.
4. Fayyad, U.; Piatetsky-Shapiro, G.; Smyth, P. The KDD Process for Extracting Useful Knowledge from Volumes of Data. *Commun. ACM* **1996,** *39* (11), 27–34.
5. Fayyad, U.; Piatetsky-Shapiro, G.; Smyth, P. From Data Mining to Knowledge Discovery in Databases. *AI Mag.* **1996,** *17* (3), 37–37.
6. Watson, H. J. Tutorial: Big Data Analytics: Concepts, Technologies, and Applications. *CAIS* **2014,** *34,* 65.
7. Chen, C. P.; Zhang, C. Y. Data-Intensive Applications, Challenges, Techniques and Technologies: A Survey on Big Data. *Inf. Sci.* **2014,** *275,* 314–347.
8. Wu, X.; Zhu, X.; Wu, G. Q.; Ding, W. Data Mining with Big Data. *IEEE Trans. Knowl. Data Eng.* **2014,** *26* (1), 97–107.
9. Safavian, S. R.; Landgrebe, D. A Survey of Decision Tree Classifier Methodology. *IEEE Trans. Syst. Man Cybern.* **1991,** *21* (3), 660–674.
10. Rokach, L.; Maimon, O. Top-Down Induction of Decision Trees Classifiers-a Survey. *IEEE Trans. Syst. Man, Cybern. Part C (Appl. Rev.)* **2005,** *35* (4), 476–487.
11. Han, J.; Pei, J.; Kamber, M. *Data Mining: Concepts and Techniques*; Elsevier, 2011.
12. Loh, W. Y.; Shih, Y. S. Split Selection Methods for Classification Trees. *Stat. Sin.* **1997,** *7,* 815–840.

13. Rahman, M. G.; Islam, M. Z. Missing Value Imputation Using Decision Trees and Decision Forests by Splitting and Merging Records: Two Novel Techniques. *Knowledge-Based Syst.* **2013,** *53,* 51–65.
14. Song, Y. Y.; Ying, L. U. Decision Tree Methods: Applications for Classification and Prediction. *Shanghai Arch. Psychiatry* **2015,** *27* (2), 130.
15. Phyu, T. N. Survey of Classification Techniques in Data Mining. *Proc. Int. Multi Conf. Eng. Comput. Sci.* **2009,** *1,* 18–20.
16. Dehuri, S.; Ghosh, A. Revisiting Evolutionary Algorithms in Feature Selection and Nonfuzzy/Fuzzy Rule Based Classification. *Wiley Interdisciplin. Rev.: Data Min. Knowl. Discov.* **2013,** *3* (2), 83–108.
17. Ibrahim, D. An Overview of Soft Computing. *Procedia Comput. Sci.* **2016,** *102,* 34–38.
18. Ovaska, S. J.; VanLandingham, H. F.; Kamiya, A. Fusion of Soft Computing and Hard Computing in Industrial Applications: An Overview. *IEEE Trans. Syst. Man Cybern. Part C (Appl. Rev.)* **2002,** *32* (2), 72–79.
19. Che, D.; Safran, M.; Peng, Z. From Big Data to Big Data Mining: Challenges, Issues, and Opportunities. In *International Conference on Database Systems for Advanced Applications*; Springer: Berlin, Heidelberg, 2013, April; pp 1–15.
20. Gahi, Y.; Guennoun, M.; Mouftah, H. T. Big Data Analytics: Security and Privacy Challenges. In *2016 IEEE Symposium on Computers and Communication (ISCC)*; IEEE, 2016, June; pp 952–957.
21. Bhatt, C.; Dey, N.; Ashour, A. S., Eds. *Internet of Things and Big Data Technologies for Next Generation Healthcare,* 2017.
22. Tan, W.; Blake, M. B.; Saleh, I.; Dustdar, S. Social-Network-Sourced Big Data Analytics. *IEEE Internet Comput.* **2013,** *5,* 62–69.
23. Katal, A.; Wazid, M.; Goudar, R. H. Big Data: Issues, Challenges, Tools and Good Practices. In *2013 Sixth International Conference on Contemporary Computing (IC3)*; IEEE, 2013, August; pp 404–409.
24. Chen, H.; Chiang, R. H.; Storey, V. C. Business Intelligence and Analytics: From Big Data to Big Impact. *MIS Q.* **2012,** *36* (4).
25. Akter, S.; Wamba, S. F. Big Data Analytics in E-commerce: A Systematic Review and Agenda for Future Research. *Electron. Markets* **2016,** *26* (2), 173–194.
26. Chen, F.; Deng, P.; Wan, J.; Zhang, D.; Vasilakos, A. V.; Rong, X. Data Mining for the Internet of Things: Literature Review and Challenges. *Int. J. Distrib. Sens. Netw.* **2015,** *11* (8), 431047.
27. Raghupathi, W.; Raghupathi, V. Big Data Analytics in Healthcare: Promise and Potential. *Health Inf. Sci. Syst.* **2014,** *2* (1), 3.
28. Sun, J.; Reddy, C. K. Big Data Analytics for Healthcare. In *Proceedings of the 19th ACM SIGKDD International Conference on Knowledge Discovery and Data Mining*; ACM, 2013 August; pp 1525–1525.
29. Atzori, L.; Iera, A.; Morabito, G. The Internet of Things: A Survey. *Comput. Netw.* **2010,** *54* (15), 2787–2805.
30. Li, S.; Da Xu, L.; Zhao, S. The Internet of Things: A Survey. *Inf. Syst. Front.* **2015,** *17* (2), 243–259.
31. Gubbi, J.; Buyya, R.; Marusic, S.; Palaniswami, M. Internet of Things (IoT): A Vision, Architectural Elements, and Future Directions. *Future Gen. Comput. Syst.* **2013,** *29* (7), 1645–1660.

32. Marjani, M.; Nasaruddin, F.; Gani, A.; Karim, A.; Hashem, I. A. T.; Siddiqa, A.; Yaqoob, I. Big IoT Data Analytics: Architecture, Opportunities, and Open Research Challenges. *IEEE Access* **2017**, *5*, 5247–5261.
33. Roberts, C. M. Radio Frequency Identification (RFID). *Comput. Secur.* **2006**, *25* (1), 18–26.
34. Zhu, Q.; Wang, R.; Chen, Q.; Liu, Y.; Qin, W. IoT Gateway: Bridging Wireless Sensor Networks into Internet of Things. In *2010 IEEE/IFIP International Conference on Embedded and Ubiquitous Computing*; IEEE, 2010 December; pp 347–352.
35. Mainetti, L.; Patrono, L.; Vilei, A. Evolution of Wireless Sensor Networks Towards the Internet of Things: A Survey. In *SoftCOM 2011*, 19th International Conference on Software, Telecommunications and Computer Networks; IEEE, 2011 September; pp 1–6.
36. Yick, J.; Mukherjee, B.; Ghosal, D. Wireless Sensor Network Survey. *Comput. Netw.* **2008**, *52* (12), 2292–2330.
37. Lee, I.; Lee, K. The Internet of Things (IoT): Applications, Investments, and Challenges for Enterprises. *Bus. Horiz.* **2015**, *58* (4), 431–440.
38. Botta, A.; De Donato, W.; Persico, V.; Pescapé, A. Integration of Cloud Computing and Internet of Things: A Survey. *Future Gener. Comput. Syst.* **2016**, *56*, 684–700.
39. Hall, L. O.; Chawla, N.; Bowyer, K. W. Decision Tree Learning on Very Large Data Sets. In *SMC'98 Conference Proceedings*. 1998 IEEE International Conference on Systems, Man, and Cybernetics (Cat. No. 98CH36218, Vol. 3); 1998, October; pp 2579–2584.
40. Chan, P. K.; Stolfo, S. J. On the Accuracy of Meta-Learning for Scalable Data Mining. *J. Intell. Inf. Syst.* **1997**, *8* (1), 5–28.
41. Andrzejak, A.; Langner, F.; Zabala, S. Interpretable Models from Distributed Data via Merging of Decision Trees. In *2013 IEEE Symposium on Computational Intelligence and Data Mining (CIDM)*; IEEE, 2013, April; pp 1–9.
42. Strecht, P.; Mendes-Moreira, J.; Soares, C. Merging Decision Trees: A Case Study in Predicting Student Performance. In *International Conference on Advanced Data Mining and Applications*; Springer, Cham, 2014, December; pp 535–548.
43. Perera, C.; Ranjan, R.; Wang, L.; Khan, S. U.; Zomaya, A. Y. Big Data Privacy in the Internet of Things Era. *IT Prof.* **2015**, *17* (3), 32–39.
44. Behera, R. K.; Naik, D.; Rath, S. K.; Dharavath, R. Genetic Algorithm-Based Community Detection in Large-Scale Social Networks. *Neural Comput. Appl.* **2019**, 1–17.
45. Behera, R. K.; Rath, S. K.; Jena, M. Spanning tree based community detection using min-max modularity. *Proc. Comput. Sci.* **2016**, *93*, 1070-1076.
46. Gavankar, S. S.; Sawarkar, S. D. Eager decision tree. In *2nd International Conference for Convergence in Technology (I2CT)*, 2017, pp. 837–840.
47. Liu, D. S.; Fan, S. J. A Modified Decision Tree Algorithm Based On Genetic Algorithm for Mobile User Classification Problem. *Sci. World J.* **2014**.
48. Wang, X.; Liu, X.; Pedrycz, W.; Zhang, L. Fuzzy Rule Based Decision Trees. *Pattern Recognit.* **2015**, *48*(1), 50–59.
49. Borgelt, C., Höppner, F., & Klawonn, F. *Guide to Intelligent Data Analysis*. Springer-Verlag London Limited.

50. Song, I. Y.; Zhu, Y. (2016). Big Data and Data Science: What Should we Teach? *Expert Syst.* **2016,** *33*(4), 364–373.
51. Zhou, J., Cao, Z., Dong, X.; Vasilakos, A. V. Security and Privacy for Cloud-based IoT: Challenges. *IEEE Commun. Mag.* **2017,** *55*(1), 26–33

CHAPTER 5

THE EMERGING ROLE OF THE INTERNET OF THINGS (IoT) IN THE BIOMEDICAL INDUSTRY

AMRIT SAHANI and SUSHREE BIBHUPRADA B. PRIYADARSHINI[*]

Computer Science and Information Technology, Institute of Technical Education and Research, Siksha 'O' Anusandhan, Deemed to be University, Bhubaneswar 751030, India

[*]*Corresponding author. E-mail: bimalabibhuprada@gmail.com*

ABSTRACT

This chapter summarizes and conveys the advancement of Internet of things (IoT) in the medical industry and also summarizes the network architectures conjointly with medical industry demand as well as various trends and phases in the organized provinces of the health sector to the community development. In this connection, IoT involves elegant and fashionable objects and the most crucial building section in the advancement of virtual cyber environment and mechanism that is entirely controlled and tracked through employing various Internet devices followed by uniting global computer network and its users. The IoT splits into numerous applications and software provinces starting from the range of home appliances to the very well-accepted healthcare production. Moreover, the IoT revolution is reshaping the modern health industry with aspiring profitable money—making a communal revolution with the involvement of technology. Further, this chapter throws light on the working of IoT, its architecture, and its implementation in healthcare units such as electrocardiogram (ECG) monitoring, glucose level sensing, body temperature tracking, and wheelchair handling.

5.1 INTRODUCTION

In the recent last few years of the human history, life sciences and its advancements have set exceptional representation and advancement in various fields and much directed in the path of Internet of things (IoT)-based devices that are not only helping the people but also serving its role to the patients, doctors, and the entire industry.[1] Life science and the pharmaceutical industry have seen a traditionalist rate of adopting the use of new technology; however, its demand has been pacified in the last few years. IoT in recent years has gained faith in real-time diagnosis, effective monitoring, and many other preventive measures and other long-standing chronic conditions where a need for proactive action is most binding and much more active sessions that are practicable with the aid of IoT implanting different sensors and smart gadgets in the surroundings to keep the track of real-time data.[2,3]

5.1.1 BRIEF OVERVIEW OF INTERNET OF THINGS (IoT)

The IoT is a structure of mixed and winded computing, computational devices, both are operated mechanically and electrically. It also involves digitized machines, specified objects, animals, humans, and people, which are equipped with different and apparent identifiers and have the capacity to transfer information, resources, and valuable data over an integrated network without any man-to-man or man/human along with computer interaction directly.[4] There are processes that integrate to form the IoT. The IoT is a prominent topic of techno-management and socializing skills with great economic importance and time reduction in various ways for people across the globe. Starting from the consumer and durable goods to other industrial components, its usages also penetrates to the everyday objects.

All the devices of the IoT remain connected with the Internet and receive information from the Internet. With a statistical powerful data analytics, it has the strength to endure the transformation of the type of work we are involved in and takes out insightful information of real-time data track as most of the information is stored in a cryptic way over the servers. The information stored in the servers is matched with a design of a graph. Any abrupt disorder in the graph reprimands the user regarding the unusual activity. This unusual disorder helps a lot to the doctors pertaining to the medical industry as the amount of unusual activity warns the doctor regarding the patient's health and substantial care is being taken for the respective patients. IoT devices also keep a track of the heart rate and the other body activities of the patients and inform the doctors, and if any disorders are taken into consideration first, they are treated with utmost care. Along with analytics, the IoT increases considerable questionnaire hurdles that stand in the path of the potential benefits.[4]

All the time, the devices are connected to the Internet to receive information from the servers. There is always a potential risk of attention from dishonest customers and the considerable risk of hacking of such device; concerns about surveillance and fears concerning privacy and many such threats have gathered public attention. Challenges in the technical field, privacy policies, and other legal challenges are under constant hindrance to the field of emerging technology.[3,4]

If an Android or an iOS operating system (mobile phone) conciliates the user by giving them a user-friendly interface to interact with the designs, databases, and connections from different parts of the world with the help of social media tools and web browsers, the users also become aware of the world from the news section available in their technological tool. Similarly, IoT in healthcare makes the same use of independence and helps out doctors, surgeons, and sometimes patient to check the smooth running of the body systems. With the help of the devices, they can keep a track record of patients' blood sugar and blood pressure levels that indirectly connect to hypertension and stress and can suggest to the patients the amount of medication possible. The entire checkups and medical claim database can be monitored by the physician through a smartphone. And yes these smart devices depend on a range and statistics of data. The information and the data are compared to the normal database—if it lies in the specified range of data, the patient is in stable condition, else if the data are unusual or outside the normal range, an alert or some kind of notifications are generated, which indirectly draws an attention toward a specific curing/treatment.[2,4]

Nowadays, such devices are being connected with the health claim to afford a base at the pharmaceutical industry at the root level of diagnosis, treatment, and rehab and therapeutic center. So an intelligent, integrated, united, and collaborated model of IoT can minimize the risk of a patient's health and can make doctors predict the consequences for future use. So smart innovations and technical gadgets with the use of artificial intelligence (AI), big data, and others can be gripped in the healthcare context, which can address various IoT and e-health across various environment, facilitate the growth of healthy society, and thus improve the socioeconomic development in terms of sustainable development and provide some path for the next-generation research on IoT-based healthcare.

IoT splits categorically into four distinct parts:

- sensors/devices
- user connectivity
- data processing and collection and mining of data
- a user interface

5.1.1.1 SENSORS

This comes to existence as building blocks for IoT and could be as simple as reading of any information or data from somewhere else. Sensors/data collectors packed into a single unit can be used as a proper device, which detects every stable condition of the environment through which the information gets traced.[2-4]

5.1.1.2 CONNECTIVITY

This stage plays a vital role between the device and the user. The device is connected with cloud computing and wireless technology in combination with Bluetooth, Wi-Fi, Ethernet, Internet, etc. By choosing the capacity of networking and the reliable strength of the wireless technology, IoT applications/devices can be categorically divided.[4]

5.1.1.3 DATA PROCESSING/DATA MINING

As the name suggests, this phase collects data from the environment or the data that get fed on the devices and software gets down to preprocess it with the use of algorithms or fixing them in an assigned range. After the modification, it is passed on to the users who actually use the benefits of IoT.[4]

5.1.1.4 USER INTERFACE

The information collected and reformed are made useful to the customers who really enjoy the value. Depending upon the information received, further actions are made easier pertaining to automatic or manual approach depending on the strength of the IoT device.

5.1.2 BACKGROUND STUDY

With the advanced growth of information technologies along with communication advancements such as Bluetooth Low Energy and 3G/4G/5G, substantial growth of the Internet as well as its users have given a hike to an everlasting advanced technical device called the IoT.[4] In IoT-based devices, contactless data collecting and information collection and analyzing of the retrieved information that are the fundamental concepts for delivering the best man-aided services in a more effective clear and transparent way are there is a motive to achieve the systems more quickly.[5–7]

Among all these advanced aids and services, the advancement of IoT in the medical industry is the most positive and important direction and, therefore, focuses more on the industrial and government services. A healthcare system is mostly exploited for the utilization of data collection, storage of data, and information needed for the modern nursing activities through the use of modern information and communication tools. With the help of contactless technology and efficiency kept forward by the data retrieval techniques on IoT objects, many systems have been developed promptly to serve mankind and these smart objects are always in constant support to the pharmacy market. The issuance of system security and the privacy of the patients are considered at the topmost level. This agenda is the main focus by the researchers, developers, and various other existing government/private entities.[5,7]

The ability to show up patient privacy and security of the system is always vulnerable. There are times where patients' privacy may not be taken into consideration where the resource/information is collected, analyzed, and stored in the information system database of any particular hospital where the lateral is being cured. Based on the observance, there are some major principles that are included in the data cleansing and processing:

  i) Data cleansing can be used and processed for genuine and lawful uses.

ii) Unauthorized ways and malpractice measures have been treated with the utmost scrutiny.
iii) Responsibility should be measured.
iv) Agreement for the processing of data should be done at the prior level.
v) Consent regarding privacy and protection should be dealt with as early as possible.
vi) Sufficient information must be shared for which the information and research are being utilized.

So in this chapter, we are representing and dealing with a robust study on IoT-based healthcare units and medical support systems in which the environmental objects essential for sensing are employed in the body of the patients to keep a track on high-quality assurance for building a healthy environment.

5.2 REPORTS AND APPROACHES USED

5.2.1 REPORTS

According to various reports, the adoption of the latest technology and IoT may bring an exceptional advancement for the mankind in the next few years and its applications have also changed the lives of many in the last few years as well. The current operational hospitals use efficient ways and they have done a great advancement in managing the day-to-day operations in the clinics and also keep a track of the e-health of different hospitalized patients. The researchers are currently trying to dig deep into the data received from all the healthcare devices and are finding out an excellent meaningful pattern of the data and are analyzing the amount of drug control and the type of the pattern of treatment and various other protective measures that can be taken in order to safeguard the life of the patients and other people living in the environment.[8,9]

It is a good point that can be noted that the global industry for the e-healthcare has increased its way and is on with bouncing trends. A complete understanding of the current scenario of the IoT-enabled different wearables and accessories is the most useful information for the research in future purpose, particularly, the different aspects of the wearable devices and the unity of all joining with information technology authorized with the sensors.

In summary, the chapter enlightens on the following works:

i) Study and research on different devices support IoT, including the hardware and software, as other technologies used for communication and other platforms are needed for the sustainability of the healthcare services;
ii) Comparing different devices used and other existing IoT wearables that can be used for IoT healthcare devices;
iii) Finding out the challenges associated with the healthcare field;
iv) Analysis of the information obtained in this study.

5.2.2 METHODS USED

This part makes us introduce the basic and rudimentary concepts of the IoT architecture and the communication that are embedded in the devices to the proposed healthcare support system, which includes an authentication and registration module.

5.2.2.1 COMMUNICATION SCENARIO IN THE TARGETED FIELD

This part of the chapter introduces the audience about the communication system for the scenario on target, that is, management of the patients and the rehabilitation in which the environmental sensors are fixed and the device's sensors are fitted on the field and the body of the patient. There are three important components in the field of communication and healthcare.

i. A nursing server usually present in the back end,
ii. A mobile gateway (handled mostly by the nursing back end in charge persons),
iii. IoT devices, smart gadgets, etc.

The devices used for gathering information and collecting several environmental consistencies as healthcare are very sensitive and are highly vulnerable to any minute change in the regular environment. All the data from the patients and the information collected get operated and are under constant visualization with the caretaker through a mobile gateway. The information from highly sophisticated machines like electrocardiography, electroencephalography, and electromyography and the blood pressure is also retrieved in a similar way under constant surveillance demanding on the condition of the patient. The back-end team of nurses can regularly check the patient's condition through this without particularly visiting the patients. Figure 5.1 shows a scenario of the registration phase. More the information, more accurate will be the treatment services delivered.

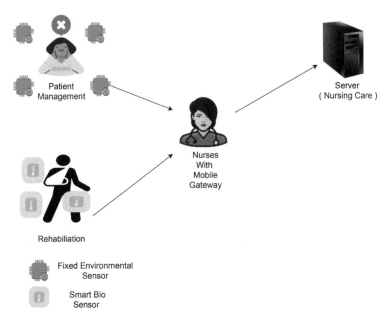

FIGURE 5.1 Phases of registration.

5.2.2.2 IoT-BASED NURSING SYSTEM

This part proposes the nursing unit of the support system in which the IoT and other smart devices that are run with the help of IoT help in providing the patients with a suitable continuous care environment. The surgeons use their mobile gateway, which is portable, lightweight, and easy to carry to retrieve the data from the smart objects. All the data information collected so far get stored in the servers at the back end (generally access is not granted to the general public). Then the information shared is under constant updating with the doctors in charge and necessity steps are taken when there is an unusual change in the graph or other eccentric information also attracts special attention to the patients. Figure 5.2 illustrates a scenario of user authenticatiion.[10,11]

The Emerging Role of the Internet of Things (IoT) 137

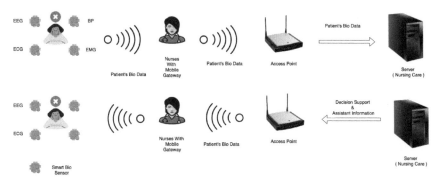

FIGURE 5.2 Phases of authentication.

Basically, a system includes two parts:

A) Registration phase
B) Authentication phase

In the registration phase, the security and other threats to the information, the persons to whom the information is shared, and other entities to which the information is passed on are taken into consideration, that is, the information retrieved from the devices are passed through the gateway and eventually to the back-end servers over a cryptic way. After a series of information passing through authentication process, phase id gets deployed just to ensure the security checks so that data are easily exchanged and shared in the most secure way. The support system is able to settle security achievements while ensuring the authentication among various devices across each step. Further, resisting any vulnerable threats to the systems from outside is made to securely establish a good authentication between the registration phase and the phase of authentication and also check no other persons other than the assigned people to use the system.

Instruments in hospitals that can be used for:

- Living in a world where we are constantly supported by waves of electronic devices oozing from the gadgets we use on a daily basis.
- The IoT objects allow us to be more at ease as the connected devices with the Internet communication help us in making our life more comfortable.

- All the gadgets have a basic principle of collecting information, cleansing the missing data and analyzing the shared data coming from the sensors so that they can draw a beautiful pattern of the received information and can be used to predict the outcomes in the near future.
- Any changes in the values in future can remind the people of the unusual behavior.[10,11]

Here are some advantages when we take into consideration of health management and healthcare systems.

The health system makes the most profit from such design and analysis patterns and different graph plots regarding the sensitive areas, including heart rate, pulse rate, sleep monitoring, the number of calories burnt, and the additional amount of proteins and minerals required for a human to remain healthy and fit. Patients do not need to carry the urine sample to the doctor; sensors can log the body movement patterns and the other sensors in the bathroom can predict the following designs depending upon the time of water usage and the amount of water consumed. A physician can set a fixed amount of running distances for the patients suffering from sugar and also people having an excess of cholesterol.[10,11]

5.2.2.3 MONITORING IN-PATIENTS' HEALTH

Sensors track the records of patients and monitor the activities of the persons from the time they arrive in a hospital or can be tracked even before from their home with the use of smart environment assembled at their home. This helps the surgeons who look into the healthcare as they get a tracking activity of the patient for the last few days and they suggest the best medication quickly without any delay, whereas if they do not have a track record of the patient, then doctors, surgeons check the entire body and end up with certain tests so in this way the medication gets a couple of days late.[12,13]

But what happens when they are in the hospital; so there must be a device to monitor the health in the treatment center. Hospital beds are also the perfect choice and preferentially sensors must be placed in the closest propinquity to detect things faster and quicker. The use of smart devices can also help the patients to order their daily meals and juices at just one tap and patients can easily know their surgeons and nurse team and manage the temperature of the room without disturbing other people in the ward. Figure 5.3 shows the scenario of working of IoT in healthcare units.

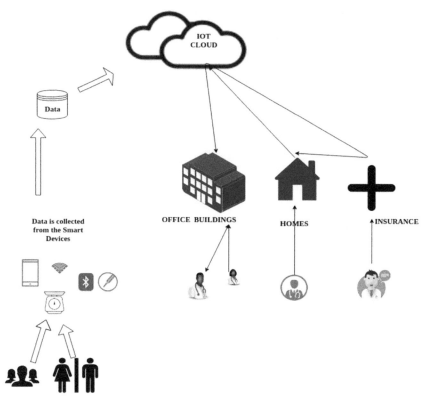

FIGURE 5.3 Working of IoT in healthcare units.

5.2.2.4 OPTIMIZING CARE

A hospital is a place full of people and is always a busy place with thousands of patients coming and leaving on a daily basis. In such a busy place of patients and doctors, expensive medical equipment may be present. Sometimes, it may happen that patients can miss the right medication and the resources sought become useless; so the assignment of beds to the respective patients must be done in a careful and planned so as not to put a danger to the life of any patient and systematic assignments also ensure a carefree environment of patients. The doctors find it more convenient for their daily checkups.[14,15] So an autobed system helps the doctors from this case. It uses a complex real-time algorithm just to check the real-time availability of the beds with the help of sensors attached to the beds. The algorithm uses different devices of radio frequency and figures out of the empty bed and which bed to be allotted for an incoming patient.

It also checks the patient's condition and if possible allocates the nearest bed to the most critical patient in coming to the hospital, which is decided by the surgeons in charge over there.

So these are some of the ways in which IoT is used in a constructive way in the field of the healthcare system.

Other institutes and organizations are working on the concepts of computer vision for deep learning and also track the natural body movement recognition. Further, the devices also record the presence of staffs and assess the safety risks of the environment to control the temperature, noise, and brightness of the room, so these engines use AI models to predict the moods and behavior of the patients by knowing the environment in which they want to live. And the doctors also look into their patients' behavior and treat them to their same fulfillment. Figure 5.4 illustrates a scenario of indoor GPS for hospital. Similarly, Figure 5.5 shows a scenario of monitoring and tracking in healthcare sector.

In the hospitals, there must be attention to be paid to every detail to the inventory and checklist items present here and there as well as to the maintenance. IoT could help a lot in these areas to keep an eye on the minute details, which would else need a lot of man working over them. So the real-time location system can be used to help people locate the tracking and the staffs can use it for the management of the medical types of equipment, patients and different types of environments. The location data may vary as this data is not to be captured from the satellite real-time data but rather it detects the location generated from the devices in the hospital. It works similarly the real-time location detection with the real-time surveillance of people using the devices.

Witnessing a great impact in the field of healthcare, a generation is heading toward a new revolution. When mankind and human life are heading toward a destination of the well-being of the people, the extended healthy life of the people is bringing a challenge to the healthcare industrial domain. Healthcare industry and all the rest of the organizations tied up into the health domain must alter their tools of supervision of health monitoring so that they do not get inundated with a year-long data. So the implementation and the use of IoT are the best possible solution to these problems. Before bringing on with the implementations of IoT devices and their substantial role in the healthcare industry, there is a briefing on healthcare. The biomedical industry is such a huge, complex, interconnected system that uses IoT appearing to be never-ending. Starting from the monitoring of the remote personal healthcare to sensors embedded in the health devices, other smart building facilities, and smart pills, it not only keeps the patient's health well but also has an improvisation to the traditional care system. IoT focuses on the monitoring of the patient's health, tracking and coordinating, and observance of other records.

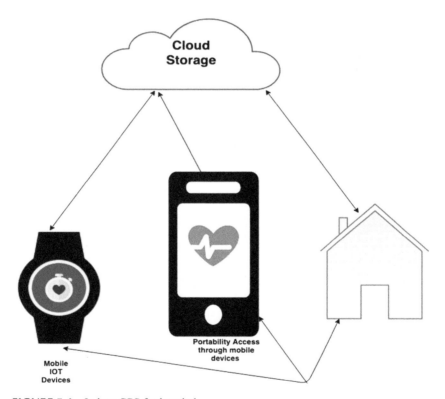

FIGURE 5.4 Indoor GPS for hospital.

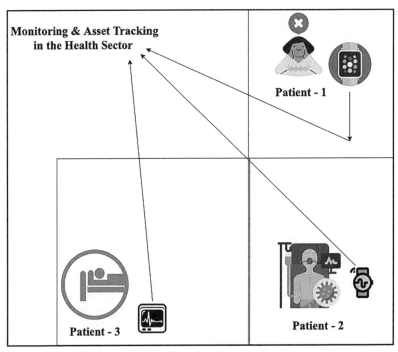

FIGURE 5.5 Monitoring and ensnaring in healthcare sector.

The foundation stone of IoT application started its way from the records of patient's health and shaping it to a way of computerized monitored electronic health record, which the industry peculiarly calls the e-health data. These online-generated data and records have become prominent in the last few years, while the demand for maintaining the patient's history over pen and paper becomes insignificant. The use of the electronic devices assures the advancement mutualism in the field of medical care. It also smoothens the interaction between the patients and the families and reduces the inconsistency in the ladder of efficiency.

5.2.2.5 TELE-HEALTH

The use of the electronic mass media and data and other communication-advanced machinery, and equipment has cut the rope of distant clinical healthcare.

Various ways of the implementation of telehealth are as follows:

A. **Video live:** The interaction between the end user and any physician or any particular hospital with the use of smart devices and an Internet connection is called video live. Video telecasting can be used for both the treatment as well as the diagnosis.[16,17]
B. **Save the records:** The recorded health history of the particular patients are stored in the cloud services and can be retrieved to and fro from any other hospital or doctors for future reference. It communicates all the illness and the diagnosis done on the patients and the doctors examining during the treatment. It creates a good reference for the next surgeon for the immediate steps to be taken.
C. **Monitoring the patient remotely:** The health of the patient and the data collected from every subject each from a different location are then sent to the server present in a different location. This way is not profusely used but still, the health provider can keep across the people using its smart device and predict the outcomes of their health referencing to the average human health.

5.2.2.6 M-HEALTH

By leaps and bound in the telecom sector, our smartphone industry has a splendid increase in the market cap. Moreover, its presence has penetrated the healthcare industry influencing the positivity and makes the use of smart health devices more conveniently. Applications bound to the mobile devices can target a set of audience and keep them announcing the updates through the Internet and other communication technology.[18–20] The integration of the old record system along with the IoT can create a personal experience of healthcare solutions. Applications can influence the targets through personal messages, timely notifications or systematic mail generations, or any other desirable options that the clients choose according to its comfort and substance used. The integration of IoT along with the e-healthcare record system can provide a practical solution to numerous problems that are as follows:

- Connecting any wearable or any portable device to the cloud systems to store information to the databases scattered over the Internet
- Also helps to analyze the collected information across all the devices that are connected mutually in a peer-to-peer network

- Makes charts, graphs, and diagrams based on some prediction algorithms that are collected with the help of all devices
- Monitoring the health of the patient through live streaming
- In the case of any abrupt discontinuous patterns in the graphs, which may lead to unstable conditions, they are also reported to the nearby family members or can be informed to the doctors.

5.2.2.7 CONNECTED MEDICAL/HEALTH DEVICES

The wearable devices, portable devices, and monitoring devices that are helping out the patients are nowadays a popular stock in the market. Such devices, including the pumps of insulin (used for insulin pump cardiac monitoring devices, BP machines [blood pressure checking device]), CPAP machines, and some other oxygen tank pipes, are also being used together to ensure proper surveillance and care for the patients giving them timed punctuality.[12,19,20]

Moreover, some device manufacturing units offer an online platform to enable the storage and transfer and the showcasing of health data and also allows the interoperability across different devices and platforms that would help the industry to grow and have a deep impact on the research and paperwork that are going on relentlessly. IoT devices can help the clients to stay in a healthy environment, make the patients tend toward the path of a quick recovery, and also treat them without moving to a medical center. It can save money for both the institutes/organizations and produce the results in a quicker way along with the treatment; interconnectivity can also provide an easy collection of data and management of all the assets and remote control device management. Figure 5.6 shows a scenario of capability of various IoT devices.[18–20]

5.3 SMART HOSPITALS

The word seems to be quite peculiar. So continuing in the queue of advancement and other facilities opted by the IoT is indeed induced by the clients everywhere. Smart hospitals are special versions of the modern hospitals but with a different approach of optimization, design, built-in structure, and different other clinical processes that use digitized infrastructure collateral with interconnected objects specifying the process of automation and built on the rudimentary model of AI and IoT.[18,20]

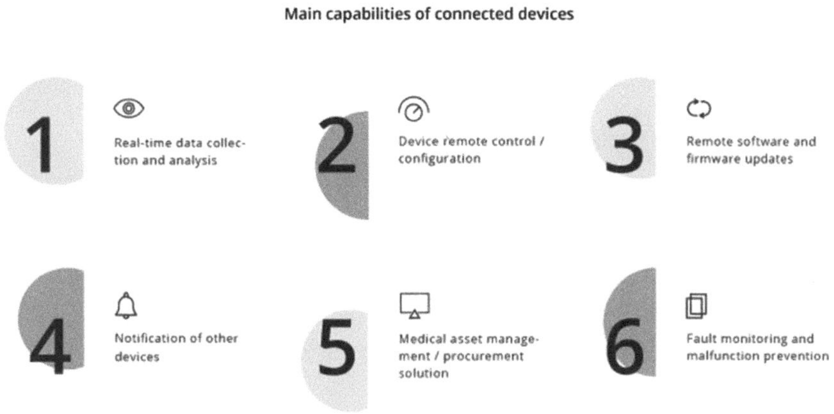

Main capabilities of connected devices

1. Real-time data collection and analysis
2. Device remote control / configuration
3. Remote software and firmware updates
4. Notification of other devices
5. Medical asset management / procurement solution
6. Fault monitoring and malfunction prevention

FIGURE 5.6 Capabilities of IoT devices.

The smart hospital is a working model and is now used by various industries for a daily checkup of workers working there and also in some parts of the country on a trial basis.

They work on some basic principles that are as follows:

a. Collection of data,
b. Taking out different meanings and stories from the data,
c. Having access to the data to specific groups so that they can decide the smartest initiative to the action taken.

The knowledge taken from the data helps to know the patient condition, analyze the future consequences of the particular disease, and thus steps are taken by which it can be prevented. The smart hospitals make the smart decision of any tasks related to clinical operations and the patient favorability.

5.3.1 OPERATIONS EFFICIENCY

It can be achieved by making the systems automated and implementing the smart machine tools to have improvised maintenance and superficial solutions toward the management.

5.3.2 CLINICAL EFFICIENCY TASKS

It is always the concerned topic to discuss on and improve the surgeon's efficiency of work done by the nurses.[20] It also ensures the monitoring of patients and patient involvement.

5.3.3 PATIENT WELL-BEING

The centricity for the patients in the smart hospitals helps us to improve the standards of patient's experience, building the smart hospital rooms with voice-simulated experience to call on the nurses or to control the tempera.ture of the room and controlling the lighting of the room.

Figure 5.7 describes the important capabilities of connected devices.

Among the main capabilities of connected devices we can mention

A — Building connected rooms

B — Electronic medical record management

C — Smartphone-based assistant applications for caregivers

D — Smart consoles to allow patients to track their treatment process and communicate with clinicians or the world

E — Integration of monitoring devices with analytics software throughout a hospital to provide physicians with greater visibility into patient's vitals

F — Control of the building's environmental characteristics, such as temperature, humidity, pressure, noise, etc.

G — Pharmacy inventory management and other tagging technologies

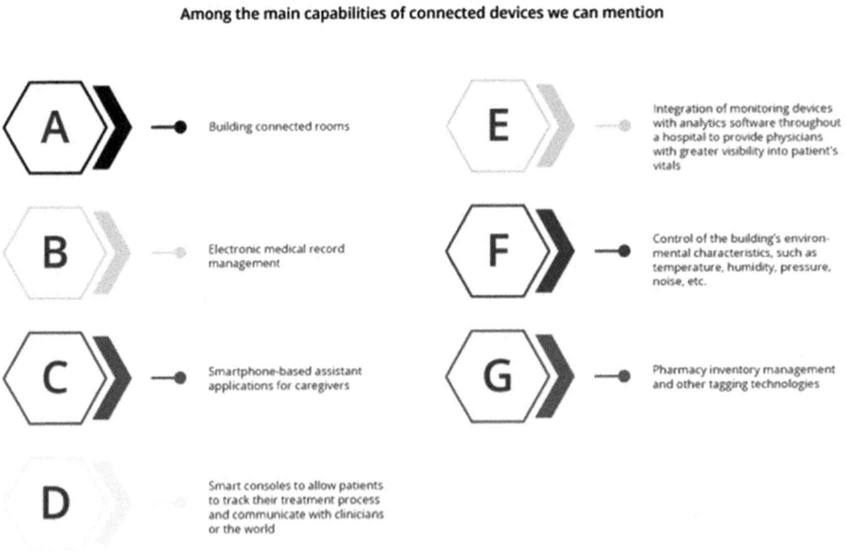

FIGURE 5.7 Major capabilities of connected devices.

Other small-scale devices that also make the lives of the patient more comfortable are as follows:

  A. **Hearables (audio/challenging devices)**—These are some of the new aids for the people suffering from ear ailment or having a

low-audible rate. These devices operate as hearing aids, which on wearing allow hearing at a clear rate. The device filters the sound and adds some layered features to the real world.
B. **Ingestible sensors**—These represent the sensors used for monitoring any irregularities in the body of the patient. They are the small bean-sized sensors that monitor the medication in the body of the patient. This application helps a diabetic patient and regulates the amount of sugar present in the healthy body and if any irregular behavior might quote an early medication and it also warns to take proper and immediate actions.
C. **Moodles**—These are the devices that enhance the mood and helps in supervising the mood. These are the devices that are mounted on the head and these devices continuously send low-intensity shocks or in simple words can be termed current to the brain to intensify and elevate the mood. Inspite of integrating the values of IoT and other important specifications into the health and medical domain, it would bring a lot of esteemed value for the higher age-group and patients suffering from chronic conditions and those who require a constant observation with extreme care.
D. **Swift recognition of drugs and medicine**—Prevailing from the information, we can get accustomed to the fact that a partial work in the healthcare industry can be done with the help of smart devices and IoT. However, proving the effective use of devices and their correlating diagnostics have been done; however, we introduce AI along with IoT, which can result in much better effects in the industry. So for every problem from the patient's end, we relate it to the scale of problems and develop a strategy for AI to find out a close result or an approximate optimal solution, which benefits all the environment variables in every possible fashion. According to reports, $2.5 billion and one decade of research eventually end the description of the drug development process.[18,19]

As mentioned in the section before, only 1 single entity of a drug from a bunch of 10 would go through all the necessary conditions and then reach the end users. In the present day, the world advancing with tremendous speed can neither impart such exorbitant expenses nor such prolonged time module of developing a single medicine, the chance of which reaching the market is merely 10%. Here the process of AI and IoT combines to perform a better logistical solution to enhance the drug development process. So it is here where the use of AI and some smart devices, which embedded with AI can predict the discovery of drugs in a more faster and cost-effective manner. The proponents of the techniques of AI and machine learning will escort to a time-saving supplementary discovery of drug. Reports postulate that the efficient tool for generating drug with smart inventions can make the profit making up to 100 billion in pharmaceutical industry.

Phases of drug development are as follows:

Stage 0. Overview of the literature

In this present scenario, the extensive research that gets published on a day-to-day basis can accumulate a lot of insightful knowledge to formulate a more understandable hypothesis. So it is practically impossible for mankind to read all the journals and periodical publications. Most of the authors' quote work not on a larger field but rather choose one field to describe the most efficient paperwork.

So this can be a solution to allow the machines to read all the available resources and information, documents, and even the patients to stipulate them into a single entity fact of database, which can indeed form the basis of the hypothesis to find a solution of the disease targeted.[20]

Stage 1. Target the identification for the interruption

The initial steps taken into the development of drugs are to understand the origin of a species of disease and the limit to which it resists. The ailment of a disease is important to specify the targets that are better than others, most of the cases use proteins. It is also a challenging task to implement the higher variety of information and clubbing them to find a systematic pattern; so the machine learning algorithms are there to rescue, handle, and predict the data automatically to generate the target mechanism.

Stage 2. Discovery of drug candidates

With the source of information available to the researchers, they start discovering complex elements that can interact with the target identities in the derivable pattern and result in the best possible outcomes. This stage involves the testing of millions of natural potential proteins and other available resources to see the results and also keep an eye on the side effects. The machine learning algorithms and the AI production can enhance the productivity model with the enhanced descriptors of modular and molecular structure and filter the results with the least available side effects.

Stage 3. The faster approach in medical trails

The success of the approach rests on the selection of suitable and appropriate candidates because the wrong decision may lead to the extension of trails and waste time unnecessarily and also has an effect on the increase in the demand for resources, which indirectly increases the cost of production. Algorithms of machine learning along with IoT devices can predict the best possible outcomes and can notify the researchers about the medical trails that are producing the concluding results and possibly saving the embryonic development of the drug.

Stage 4. Biomarkers identification for Treatment of the Disease

Inclusive of all conclusions, you can only treat the patients for a particular disease of which you are extremely sure for diagnosis. The biomarkers are the molecules that are present in the fluids of the human body and provide us with the supreme certainty so that whether the patient is suffering from a particular disease or not indeed by making the process cheap. The molecules can also be used to detect the headway to correct treatment and supervise the working of the drug.

Biomarkers identification involves the following steps:

- Detect the presence of a deformity as soon as possible
- Detect the risk developing from the disease and the extent to which it can harm the patient
- Detect the progress
- Detect whether the response to a particular drug will be positive toward a certain disease

Sightseeing all these improvisations and the shifts suggest that the medical and pharmaceutical industry embracing the concepts of machine learning with the touch of IoT and AI has helped a lot in screening the drugs and predicting the necessary outcomes for the drug candidates and reduces the effective cost, time of research, and development team.

5.4 CAN IOT TECHNOLOGY BE THE EXPERTISE IN THE FUTURE FOR HUMANS?

The way by which the commencement of the technology that we use in the normal routine can be held by the series of concepts of AI and the use of IoT, which are joined together to form a distinct argument. As custodian, humans will find a designated problem and allow the algorithms to find a solution. The generation will attune the target-specific compounds, diseases and find a suitable diagnosis for the same. Concluding the subsequences, the future stays in the correlation between the humans and the smart devices, so the doctors and other surgeons should have to adapt to learn and fatten the technological advancements. The future expertise remains in the combination of both medical and tech experts to find an evolution in the pharmaceutical industry and eluding some critical problems.[21–24]

Some of the challenges that should be kept and overcome for the smooth functioning of the devices working on the Internet are described in the following sections.

5.4.1 PRIVACY AND SECURITY OF DATA

The most important concern and the significant threat to the people and devices across the globe is the security concern of the information related to personal issues and information of the patient. The objective and the design of the IoT devices receive and transmit information in real time for the analysis and cleansing of data. The capital requirement for processing the information and a medium for receiving it should be designed in a way to obtain the scalability of receiving and broadcasting information to store and process the real-time data over the servers. The sources oozing from the smart devices and wearables suffer a lot of protocols and regulations, and as a result, the data are always vulnerable to threat and suffer persistent privacy norms. The information available and generated from the devices are a lot more precious to the world of cybercrime and who can easily use data from the selective patient and exploit the treatment activities or can misuse the data for any other firm.[22]

It can be used to sell or buy illegal drugs or to generate fake ID's and too can file fraudulent claims from the insurance vendors with the name of the patient or under his name and also can be used to buy expensive medicines that are of limited supply under the name of the patient. So the technology manufacturers and the hospitals should take very energetic measures to make the environment sure about the hackability. The vendors must also be careful and examine the products before cracking the deal of the products.

5.4.2 CALAMITIES

Natural calamities and disasters cause an adverse effect causing huge damage to the infrastructures, property, and other losses that can be uncountable leaving behind accountable damage to the economy. The time to recover depends on certain factors and also the damage severity caused by nature. In the case of any such calamities, the hospitals (including the smart ones) face huge damage to the infrastructure, which destroys the initial setup of Internet-originated objects and takes a long time to recover them back to rehabilitate them to their original state.[23]

5.4.3 ANALYTICS AND THE USE OF BIG DATA IN THE FIELD OF INTERNET OF THINGS (IOT)

Big data means the data that is exorbitant in nature and the summed-up information that is also enormous; the analysis of the data obtained from the source of IoT objects grants a potential to gains an endless possibility of comprehension.[24] The complication arises in a good number when dealing with the huge datasets and the possibility of analysis gets increasingly advanced. The aim of the informatics is to help the existence of life with the advanced research gathered through all the data and helps in understanding the practice of medicine and discovery of different treatment approaches. So possibilities get on with the use of IoT and storing all its data using big data tools to approach the analysis of patterns, gathering data at the different indigenous levels, and combining every insight from each base level to obtain the most stable approach in the world of healing. Later, we will penetrate different levels of informatics of health data, which are attested to different levels.

5.5 INTRODUCTION TO BIG DATA ANALYTICS AND INTERNET OF THINGS

Big data fades with any coarse definition, that is, data varies in the range of petabyte (10^{15} bytes or even more than that). Information oozed out from the IoT devices are stored over the cloud in the cluster. It uses some different approaches of storing the data into the usual database; data from the sources must have a diversion in volume, variety, values, veracity, and even velocity. Each of the V in the mechanism responds to some concept like volume tends to the huge enormous data. In this context, velocity represents the rate in which the new data is generated, veracity represents the uniqueness of the data, and value evaluates the system-generated data and checks the quality of the data taken as a reference. Data collected on all the grounds from all the devices in the domain of healthcare informatics do exhibit the qualities.[25,26] For example, datasets of the X-rays, MRI scans, and the micro-rays injected into the patients.

Velocity means the amount of data generated from the sources and which can be cleaned immediately to monitor the condition of the patient in the most effective way. Big variety deals with different sources and from which the data and information are generated and this information are of varying types, including the age and condition of the patient. The erratic condition of the situation in data handling may be possible because we are dealing with the data of a critical environment where data may be incomplete, patterns may be highly irregular, and the data can also be highly faulty (faulty data can also be seen from faulty machines and improper implantation of IoT devices in the body of the target). So these data need proper cleansing before being used. There may be some complexities generated while handling all the informatics related to the erratic data in a big volume, so it should have enough qualities to characterize the dataset. The bombardment of the data in the health informatics is being informed in bioinformation as well where the genome pattern is generated in synthetic pattern across all the subcategories. So the successful summation of the enormous data can lead to the development and improvement for the users in the health industry.

5.5.1 LEVELS IN THE DATA OF HEALTH INFORMATICS

In the subdomain of health information, there are two different levels that would be accounted: the part from where the data is gathered and the level in which the research is being proposed.[25,26]

5.5.1.1 BIOINFORMATION

The research and study in the field of bioinformatics are not taken into consideration of the old traditional healthcare domain but the research in bioinformation can be a crucial source of health information at different positions and different levels. It mainly focuses on the research analysis in the way to learn on the functioning of the human body and the environment using the molecular data. The gradual increment in the amount of the data to the developing and pertaining methods has increased and has been supervising the development of mining of data and exceptional analysis techniques that are more practical and sensitive and allowing the system to handle the big data techniques.

Data in the informatics such as expression of data in the gene and other mutation-related data that are growing continuously in a parallel mechanism with the technology are being treated with extreme care and are termed big volume of data. The issues of the big volume data can lead to extensive research and solve computational problems associated with the software. Extremely long sequences are broken down to relatively short strings, which helps in the ability to transform the analysis of bioinformatics.[25,26]

5.5.1.2 NEUROINFORMATICS

It is also a research field and a subset of each instance of data used in the devices, smart objects related to cerebral (such as MRI where such objects generate large volumes so the power of computation can keep a pace with such high-generation volume of data). Neuroinformation focuses mainly on the research work and analysis of the image and processing controls of the brain and the services provided by the brain.

As a part of learning, it also focuses on the working of the brain and the relations of the brain to other organs while emphasizing also on the information of brain images during any particular voluntary and involuntary action, so setting information for these parts constitutes the part of big data as the images, and mappings take a lot of memory.

5.5.2 CLINICAL INFORMATION

It involves the research, analysis, and the prediction of treatments that can be done to make a recovery in a fast way and help in accumulating the accuracy or the nearest correct decisions. Information is the most important as it directly works on the body of the patient and the research contains a lot of theoretical data and the health which is obtained in the aim of prediction of the clinical treatment that must be achieved. From the past and personal experience, the surgeons select the best possible treatment under the macro-volumes of data. If any new treatment or diagnosis process is obtained, then it gets added to the same macro-volume to be present for any realistic treatment or can be used as a reference to the future use.

5.6 CONCLUSIONS AND FUTURE DIRECTIONS

Basically, IoT represents a conception that considers the strong presence of technological gadgets that send and receive information over the wireless network, cable connections (mostly known as the Internet) and can have a strong connection with every other appliance, including humans to pass on the message directly or indirectly or can be united with other wireless things or objects. Healthcare data definitely reach the decision of big data and the challenging work is to sum up the aggregation and the use of data of healthcare. Overcoming these works and challenges proposed, this will need a gradual change in the cultural pattern between the users and the providers and some other parts of the industry. The biggest situation is overcoming the balance of the security threat dealt with maintaining a secured and safe system, which maintains the combination and use of data, so robust information and data challenges will report to such cases in the future where organizations' data is shared. The situation of learning the system of health and informatics related to health will serve as the guiding concept to maximize the efforts to form a solution to be used by others in finding the opportunities and following the same pattern outlined in the writings.

KEYWORDS

- ECG
- IoT
- Big data
- GPS
- AI

REFERENCES

1. Gubbi, J.; et al. Internet of Things (IoT): A Vision, Architectural Elements, and Future Directions. *Future Gen. Comput. Syst.* **2013,** *29* (7), 1645–1660.
2. Al-Fuqaha, A.; et al. Internet of Things: A Survey on Enabling Technologies, Protocols, and Applications. *IEEE Commun. Surv. Tutorials* **2015,** *17* (4), 2347–2376.
3. Malagi, M. Heath Monitoring System Based on IoT. 2017.
4. Porkodi, R.; Bhuvaneswari, V. The Internet of Things (IoT) Applications and Communication Enabling Technology Standards: An Overview. In *2014 International Conference on Intelligent Computing Applications*; IEEE, 2014.
5. Dhar, S. K.; Bhunia, S. S.; Mukherjee, N. Interference Aware Scheduling of Sensors in IoT Enabled Healthcare Monitoring System. In *2014 Fourth International Conference of Emerging Applications of Information Technology*; IEEE, 2014.
6. Catarinucci, L.; et al. An IoT-Aware Architecture for Smart Healthcare Systems. *IEEE IoT J.* **2015,** *2* (6), 515–526.
7. Doukas, C.; Maglogiannis, I. Bringing IoT and Cloud Computing Towards Pervasive Healthcare. In *2012 Sixth International Conference on Innovative Mobile and Internet Services in Ubiquitous Computing*; IEEE, 2012.
8. Khan, S. F. Healthcare Monitoring System in Internet of Things (IoT) by Using RFID. In *2017 6th International Conference on Industrial Technology and Management (ICITM)*; IEEE, 2017.

9. Paschou, M.; et al. Health Internet of Things: Metrics and Methods for Efficient Data Transfer. *Simul. Modell. Pract. Theory* **2013,** *34,* 186–199.
10. Mieronkoski, R.; et al. The Internet of Things for Basic Nursing Care—A Scoping Review. *Int. J. Nurs. Stud.* **2017,** *69,* 78–90.
11. Huang, C.-H.; Cheng, K.-W. RFID Technology Combined with IoT Application in Medical Nursing System. *Bull. Netw., Comput., Syst., Softw.* **2014,** *3* (1), 20–24.
12. McHorney, C. A.; Tarlov, A. R. Individual-Patient Monitoring in Clinical Practice: Are Available Health Status Surveys Adequate? *Qual. Life Res.* **1995,** *4* (4), 293–307.
13. Dimitrov, D. V. Medical Internet of Things and Big Data in Healthcare. *Healthcare Inf. Res.* **2016,** *22* (3), 156–163.
14. Lu, D.; Liu, T. The Application of IOT in Medical System. In *2011 IEEE International Symposium on IT in Medicine and Education,* Vol. 1; IEEE, 2011.
15. Catarinucci, L.; et al. An IoT-Aware Architecture for Smart Healthcare Systems. *IEEE IoT J.* **2015,** *2* (6), 515–526.
16. Al-Majeed, S. S.; Al-Mejibli, I. S.; Karam, J. Home Telehealth by Internet of Things (IoT). In *2015 IEEE 28th Canadian Conference on Electrical and Computer Engineering (CCECE)*; IEEE, 2015.
17. Guillén, E.; Sánchez, J.; López, L. R. IoT Protocol Model on Healthcare Monitoring. In *VII Latin American Congress on Biomedical Engineering CLAIB 2016, Bucaramanga, Santander, Colombia, October 26th–28th, 2016*; Springer: Singapore, 2017.
18. Nandyala, C. S.; Kim, H.-K. From Cloud to Fog and IoT-Based Real-Time U-Healthcare Monitoring for Smart Homes and Hospitals. *Int. J. Smart Home* **2016,** *10* (2), 187–196.
19. Catarinucci, L.; et al. An IoT-Aware Architecture for Smart Healthcare Systems. *IEEE IoT J.* **2015,** *2* (6), 515–526.
20. Jaisree, K.; et al. Smart Hospitals Using Internet of Things (IoT). *Int. Res. J. Eng. Technol. (IRJET)* **2016,** *3* (3), 1735–1737.
21. Zhang, Z.-K.; et al. IoT Security: Ongoing Challenges and Research Opportunities. In *2014 IEEE 7th International Conference on Service-Oriented Computing and Applications*; IEEE, 2014.
22. Farahani, B.; et al. Towards Fog-Driven IoT eHealth: Promises and Challenges of IoT in Medicine and Healthcare. *Future Gen. Comput. Syst.* **2018,** *78,* 659–676.
23. Lee, I.; Lee, K. The Internet of Things (IoT): Applications, Investments, and Challenges for Enterprises. *Bus. Horiz.* **2015,** *58* (4), 431–440.
24. Shang, W.; et al. *Challenges in IoT Networking via TCP/IP Architecture*; Technical Report NDN-0038. NDN Project, 2016.
25. Hersh, W. R. Medical Informatics: Improving Healthcare through Information. *JAMA* **2002,** *288* (16), 1955–1958.
26. Shim, J. Y. A Design of IoT Based Automatic Control System for Intelligent Smart Home Network. *J. Korea IoT Soc.* **2015,** *1* (1), 21–25.

CHAPTER 6

A COMPREHENSIVE SURVEY ON THE INTERNET OF THINGS (IoT) IN HEALTHCARE

DEEPAK GARG[1*], DEVENDRA KUMAR SHARMA[2], PRASHANT MANI[2], and BRAJESH KUMAR KAUSHIK[3]

[1]Department of Electronics and Communication Engineering, IIMT Engineering College, Meerut, India

[2]Department of Electronics and Communication Engineering, SRM Institute of Science and Technology, NCR Campus, Ghaziabad, India

[3]Department of Electronics and Communication Engineering, IIT-ROORKEE, Roorkee, India

*Corresponding author. E-mail: deepakgarg1985@gmail.com

ABSTRACT

In the era of fast-growing technology, Internet of things (IoT) is expanding, which involves ubiquitous Internet connectivity using standard devices, including global computing network, providing services to anyone who can access anything, anywhere, and anytime through the Internet. The IoT proves itself as a powerful domain where the fields of computer science and electronics have been merged. The IoT has autonomous control feature where the communication is made through machine to machine, which promises a great future for the technology. The IoT has extensive set of applications in heath, logistics, security, agriculture, environment, and industry.

Another IoT idea allows the invention of various sensors, gadgets, and machines, to accumulate constant information from nature. The nature of IoT being as a resource includes the tools required for a special authentication scheme that is not fully computing and energy resources. The development of IoT devices provides suitable solutions for comprehensive range of applications for smart cities, transportation, medical and healthcare, smart homes, emergency services, biomedical, etc. After introducing the IoT features, the quality and effectiveness of services are greatly achieved that provide appropriate solution for medical and healthcare services. In this chapter, we offer a comprehensive study to understand IoT technologies, applications, and smart industrial management trends in IoT-based medical and healthcare solutions. After this study, researchers highlight certain applications, statistics, and products that are derived from healthcare IoT fields.

6.1 INTRODUCTION

The Internet of things (IoT) continues its path of evolution; further possibilities are estimated by a combination with related technology approaches and concepts such as cloud computing that helps in global computing network where everything, everyplace, every service, and every network are connected with the Internet. Although the IoT mitigates the next-generation technologies that effect the complete business spectrum and unique identifiable things with their virtual representation in an Internet-like structure, its solutions provide extended benefits in the identification of smart objects and equipment with today's Internet model/infrastructure.[1] IoT is used in different environments, including healthcare institutes, homes, and aerospace.

IoT enables communication between Internetworking devices and applications, whereby physical devices communicate via the Internet. The concept of IoT began with things classified as identity communication instruments. Radio-frequency identification device (RFID) is an example of an identity communication device. Things are tagged to these devices for their identification in future and can be tracked, monitored, and controlled using remote computers connected through the Internet. The IoT has been extensively identified as a potential solution to alleviate the pressures on healthcare structures and has thus been the target of the latest research.[2-6] The concept of IoT enables, for example, GPS-based tracking, machine-to-machine (M2M) communication, communication between wearable and personal devices, and Industry 4.0. This chapter gives a comprehensive study survey for definite areas and technologies related to IoT healthcare.

IoT for healthcare: The major problem that every patient, particularly living in remote locations, found was unavailability of doctors and treatment on critical conditions. This had very dreadful consequences on people's mind about the hospitals and doctors services. Nowadays, with the implementations of new technologies by making the use of IoT devices for healthcare monitoring, these issues have been sorted to huge extent. IoT in healthcare gives the satisfaction of patients by giving more time to interact with their doctors. The usage of the IoT in healthcare is an ecosystem.

Within the overall e-health picture, more integrated approaches and advantages are sought with a role for the so-called Internet of Healthcare Things or Internet of Medical Things.

6.2 INTERNET OF THINGS

Basically, the IoT was made by the combination of two words: Internet and things, where **Internet** is a global computer network of various smart mobiles, computers, and modems, which is governed and connected by standard protocols for connected systems.

Thing is a word used to describe a physical object, an idea, and an activity, in which you do not want to be specific. Thus, IoT enables the things or objects that receive and sent the information using any path/network such as mobiles, tablets, and computers and allows the process of supervision and control via the Internet.

IoT vision: IoT is a vision where objects (watches, clocks, home devices, Healthcare instruments) become "smart" and function like living entities by sensing, communicating through embedded devices, and computing interaction with remote-controlled objects (clouds, services, processes, and applications) or persons through the Internet.

6.2.1 IoT RELATED CONCEPTS

In the future, using IoT can mix information for tasks with end users and smart things. If the purpose is the automation of all the possible procedure, including human, then the application will affect human actions directly by the actuators in the network rather than communicating information to the user. This objective is very much related to one term that is **cyber-physical system (CPS)**. Both the CPS and IoT are correlated terminology that uses for wireless, sensors, and cloud computing networks to processes for automation. The difference between both is that the CPS emphasizes hybrid systems and formal verification of dynamical systems and the IoT emphasizes communication protocols but both consider issues of privacy and security, among many others.

A **wireless sensor network (WSN)** is a network that collects data from different sensors that send its data to the central location through the network. A WSN is a technology used in IoT system for the collection of data in various applications. In any of the systems, the data collection is the first step and then that data must be analyzed and converted into shareable format with other objects. The sensors used by the WSN make the object smart and after the large procedure, these sensors help in the innovation and development in IoT system.

M2M communication is an enabling technology for IoT. The M2M is add-on tools and provides the facility to the devices to wireless access data and connection of other devices easily. The service management application is responsible for processing the data to increase the cost, productivity gains, and security. Here, the data are only integrated into machine level, because machines are not necessarily attached to the cloud stand. It is a straightforward, one-sided form of communication. The IoT application shows difference from M2M application because in IoT, the data can be achieved from different heterogeneous objects in various formats, which can be integrated without human intercession, but IoT supports the same service as M2M with more huge capabilities The IoT can be utilized in various purposes (Figure 6.1).

- Two technologies are used by the IoT systems, that is, cloud computing and edge computing.
- An IoT uses a smart object. It is not similar to the smart devices that are only Internet connected through which the interaction can enhance with an interface for predefined capabilities to chat. However, both are having the same capabilities, this is the reason of overlapping of structure. The WSN used the sensors to connect the Internet and all smart objects are not having the sensing capabilities, so this structure also overlaps because all smart objects are not included in WSN.

- With the description of M2M and ambient intelligence, the IoT provides identical but some more capabilities as these are of two different concepts.
- The CPS and IoT are two different concepts, but there is an overlap between them because CPS is used for data collection and interaction with smart objects in IoT system; actually, CPS works on actuation of objects, whereas IoT does not.

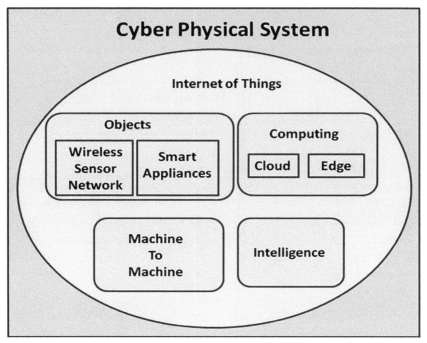

FIGURE 6.1 IoT-related concepts.

6.2.2 GENERAL FRAMEWORK OF IoT

A general framework of IoT using smart and hyper-connected devices, edge computing, and applications is shown in Figure 6.2. Computing implies computations at the device level before the computed data communications over the Internet.

6.2.3 IoT ARCHITECTURAL VIEW

A standard IoT system has four layers of architecture as shown in Figure 6.3. All these four layers are connected in a particular sequence, such that the first data are processed at the first layer and then the value transferred to next layers. A best suitable integrated value of the whole process provides the dynamic business prospects.

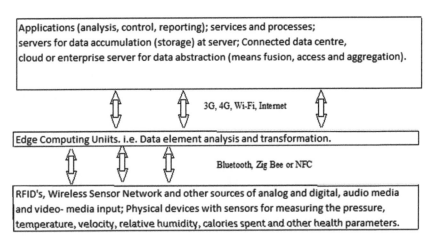

FIGURE 6.2 A general framework of IoT using smart and hyper-connected devices and applications.

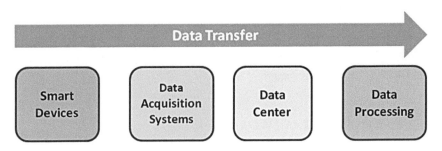

FIGURE 6.3 Four stages of IoT architecture view.[13]

- **Layer 1:** It is the first level of this architecture that consists of the development of interconnected devices such as detectors, monitors, and sensors. All these devices are used for the collection of data.

- **Layer 2:** It is the second level of this architecture that consists of various types of digital-to-analog convertors. These digital-to-analog converters are used for converting the data received from sensor and other devices that are normally in analog form. After this process, converted data are processed for further data processing.
- **Layer 3:** At the third level of this architecture preprocesses, digitized and standardized data are sent to the cloud or data center.
- **Layer 4:** At the fourth or last level of this architecture, final data are analyzed and managed at the required levels and apply the advanced analytics on the data for effective decision-making.

As per the CISCO, an IoT system has multiple levels. These levels are also known as tiers. A model enables conceptualization of a framework. A reference model can be used to depict building blocks, successive interactions, and integration. Figure 6.4 shows an IoT reference model suggested by CISCO that provides a conceptual framework for a general IoT system. This reference model consists of different seven levels.

Level 1	Physical equipment and controllers (sensors, equipment, intelligent edge nodes of various types)
Level 2	Connectivity (communication and processing units)
Level 3	Edge computing (data element analysis and transformation)
Level 4	Data accumulation (storage)
Level 5	Data abstraction (aggregation and access)
Level 6	Application (control, analysis, reporting)
Level 7	Collaboration and processes (involving people and business processes)

FIGURE 6.4 An IoT reference model suggested by CISCO that provides a conceptual framework for a general IoT system.

An architecture has the following features:

- The architecture serves as a reference in the utilization of IoT in business and service processes.
- A set of sensors are smart to capture the data, perform necessary analysis and transformation of data element as per device application framework, and contact directly to a manager.
- A set of sensor circuits is connected to a gateway possessing separate data capturing, gathering, and transmission capabilities. The data transmit from one form to another and from one end to another.

- Data routes from the gateway through the Internet and data center to the application server or enterprise server that acquires that data.
- Organization and analysis subsystems enable the services, business processes, enterprise integration, and complicated processes.

6.2.4 PARTS OF IoT SYSTEM

Dominant parts of IoT systems/devices are as follows:
  i. **Physical object** with embedded software into hardware.
  ii. **Hardware** consists of a microcontroller, firmware, sensors, control unit, actuators, and communication module.
  iii. **Communication module:** software consists of instrument APIs and instrument interface for communication over the system and middleware for creating communication stacks using 6LowPAN, CoAP, LWM2M, TPv4, and some other protocols.
  iv. **Software** for actions on messages; information and commands that the devices receive and then signal the actuators, which enables actions such as glowing LEDs and robotic hand movement.

6.3 INTERNET OF THINGS FOR HEALTHCARE

IoT involvement increases continuously in healthcare sector for enhancing the care, the result of which shows improvement in the quality of life, decreases the cost of care, and motivates the users' experience.[1] By the observation of healthcare provider, they have assured about the approximate period for cover supplies of different devices to show continuous and smooth operation. The recent healthcare trend is shown in Figure 6.5[7]. With the advancement in the cloud technologies, the electronic medical is growing and emerging with the IoT technology. Internet marketing of a technology that involves the sensor of the sensors in the field of combinations combines the Internet, the hospital, the pedestrians, and the mechanics of promotions, by promoting models of models of modern models. On the behalf of particular unique biological, cultural, behavioral, and social characteristics, the unified practice of welfare, healthcare, and individual patient support is called personal healthcare.

A Comprehensive Survey on the Internet of Things (IoT) 165

As for any topic as broad and complex as IoT, even the smaller health IoT needs to organize the information on a few selected categories. In this regard, this chapter contributes

- A comprehensive inspection of IoT-based health services and utilization.
- A comprehensive permeance into security and privacy issues around IoT healthcare solutions and proposes a model for safety.
- Discussing the key technologies that can moderate healthcare techniques on IoT basis.
- Providing benefits, which must be direct to strengthen IoT-based health-related technologies.

From the R&D section, it has been observed that the area of healthcare can be considered the primary research efforts of IoT-based healthcare based on the WSN.[9,12]

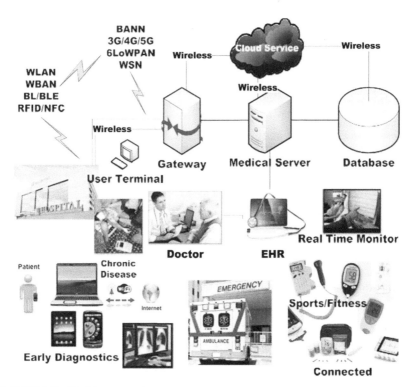

FIGURE 6.5 Healthcare trends.

6.3.1 IoT UTILITY AND APPLICATIONS FOR HEALTHCARE

The IoT-based healthcare system can be implemented in a variety of areas, including care of pediatric and old patients, medical instruments and drug control, medical information management, mobile medical care, and telemedicine.

For more clarity about this area, this chapter classifies the discussion in different facets. These aspects are generally natural and various features and much utilization can be easily increased by adding numerous services. The services and utilizations of some sections can be further explained as follows:

1. Medical information system

The IoT has much utilization in the field of information systems. The main focus of the medical information system involves recognition of doctors and patients, drug identification, medical equipment, medical records, and illness or signs. Particular utilizations include the following features:

i) Patient information management

Through the system of patient information management, the patient and doctor can share the sensitive information or medical history, which helps the doctor to diagnose the status of diseases and monitor the health of the patient from the very first day. This system also avoids the hassles that occurred in past medical systems.[10]

ii) Medication storage management

The storage management of medication can be done by RFID technology, because this management system reduces the manual or paper recording. In this the confusion about doses, similarities can be rectified by RFID and drugs can be supplied at the same time of requirement.[11]

iii) Medical emergency management

This medical emergency system is helpful in emergency cases; in some circumstances, when patients are in critical condition, then doctor can give the first aid to patient with the support of predictable and competent information depot and the investigation of RFID technology through this RFID doctor will get the identity information of patient such as name, blood group, and medical history. This will help to save valuable time for emergency patient.

iv) Blood information management

Healthcare sector is increasing by the adoption of technologies like RFID. Blood bank/information management is one of the recent developing areas of IoT. It may come as a surprise to many that due to less adequate management practices, thousands of liters of this precious resource get wasted every day across the country. Those technologies encourage efficient management in data collection.

v) Information sharing

By sharing the medical information and records, we can easily form an advanced comprehensive medical structure. Patients can also use this structure for choosing or changing their doctors or hospitals. These structures provide the full support between city and local area hospitals for sharing of information. Information sharing network is also useful for receiving the treatment guidelines of medical experts, medical training to the city and community hospitals.

2. Medical equipment and medication control

With the visualization technology of material management, we can easily observe the complete course of production, finding of medical apparatus, and medication to safeguard public medical security. The utilization of the IoT in the management and monitoring of medication and equipment includes the following aspects:

- We know that the RFID is unique for every instruments or devices. With the help of RFID tags, we can easily examine about the information of the product, so it will be the most useful way to find the counterfeit products.
- RFID tags can be used to carry out all-round observation during the complete operation of medication investigation, production, and utilizations.

3. Mobile medical and telemedicine care

i) Mobile medical care

Mobile medical care is useful for making a database for every patient or customer by observing vital signs. This type of record having maximum useful report of human body such as cholesterol, protein, weight, and fat can be analyzed in real time.

ii) Telemedicine

As per Ref. [5], a type of new medical service is telemedicine. It is merger of medical technology with the communication and computer technology. It is used to reduce the medical care cost and increase the diagnosis and medical scale. Due to the improvement of remote technology, advanced sensor has been able to completely communicate within the body sensor network[6] of patients.

Telemedicine observation has been gradually changed from focusing on increasing people's lifestyle and timely swapping of medical programs.[9]

4. Health management

i) Glucose level sensing

A set of metabolic disorders of carbohydrate metabolism characterized by higher level of sugar in blood over a long time is known as diabetes. Blood sugar observation reflects individual format of blood sugar changes and supports the schedule of activities and medication times. In Ref. [8], a medical-IoT composition approach for noninvasive sugar sensing on a real-time basis was proposed. In this approach, sensors from patient are linked with concerned healthcare providers by IPv6 connectivity.

ii) Electrocardiogram (ECG) observation

ECG observation is the main part of healthcare service. It is a graph of electrical signals or activities of the heart. The simple heart rate is measured by the ECG observation. As per Ref. [13], the utilization of the IoT to ECG observation has the potential to provide maximum useful data.

iii) Blood pressure observation

The blood pressure is frequently measured alongside the three important signs. Upper side blood pressure is the main factor causing heart attack. Hence the blood pressure must be observed regularly.[16] Equipment for blood pressure data transmission and collection over an IoT network was proposed in Ref. [17]. This equipment is composed of a blood pressure device body with a communication module.

iv) Body temperature observation

The main required part of healthcare service is body temperature monitoring. Body temperature is a decisive important sign in the maintenance of homeostasis.[19] In Ref. [20], a temperature measurement system based on a home gateway over the IoT was proposed. The user's body temperature will transmit by the home gateway with the use of infrared detection. The RFID module is the main system responsible component for temperature recording and monitoring body temperature. In Ref. [8], the concept of medical-IoT verified using a body temperature sensor was purposed.

v) Oxygen saturation observation

Pulse oximetry is used to measure the levels of oxygen in the blood. Pulse oximetry is a valuable addition to a general health observing system. The integration of the pulse oximetry with IoT is very helpful for technology-driven medical healthcare (e-health) utilizations. In Ref. [21], the potential of IoT-based pulse oximetry for a survey of CoAP-based healthcare services is discussed. In Ref. [22],[22] an IoT-optimized cost-effective pulse oximeter was proposed for remote patient monitoring. A wearable pulse oximeter using the WSN for health observing can be adapted to the IoT network.[23]

The lists of various healthcare utilizations and discussions of their required sensors, operations, and IoT associations are given in Table 6.1 and various smartphone-based healthcare apps are given in Table 6.2.

6.3.2 IoT HEALTHCARE SECURITY

The IoT technology is being adopted very vastly. In line with this development, the IoT is expected to adopt widely in the medical field and prosper through new e-health IoT devices and applications.

TABLE 6.1 Internet of Things' Utilizations for Healthcare.

Infirmity/ condition	Sensors used; operations; IoT roles/connections
Diabetes	A non-invasive opto-physiological sensor; the sensor's output is connected to the Telos B mote that converts an analog signal to a digital one; IPV6 and 6LoWPAN protocol architectures enabling wireless sensor devices for all IP-based wireless nodes.
Heart rate monitoring	Capacitive electrodes fabricated on a printed circuit board; digitized right on top of the electrode and transmitted in a digital chain connected to a wireless transmitter; BLE and Wi-Fi connect smart device through an appropriate gateway.
Body temperature monitoring	A wearable body temperature sensor; skin-based temperature measurement; WBAN connects smart devices through an appropriate gateway.
Medication management	Delamination materials and a suit of wireless biomedical sensors (touch, humidity, and CO_2); the diagnosis and prognosis of vitals recorded by wearable sensors; the global positioning system (GPS), database access, web access, RFIDs, wireless links, and multimedia transmission.
Oxygen saturation monitoring	A pulse oximeter wrist by Nonin; intelligent pulse-by-pulse filtering; ubiquitous integrated clinical environments.
Eye disorder, skin infection	Smartphone cameras; visual inspection and/or pattern matching with a standard library of images; the cloud-aided app runs on the software platform in the smartphone's SoC to drive the IoT'
Asthma chronic obstructive pulmonary disease, cystic fibrosis	A built-in microphone audio system in the smartphone; calculates the air flow rate and produces flow-time, volume-time, and flow-volume graphs; the app runs on the software platform in the smartphone's SoC to drive the IoT.
Cough detection	A built-in microphone audio system in the smartphone; an analysis of recorded spectrograms and the classification of rainforest machine learning; the app runs on the software plateform in the smartphone's SoC to drive the IoT.
Allergic rhinitis and nose-related symptoms	A built-in microphone audio system in the smartphone; speech recognition and vector machine classification; the app runs on the software platform in the smartphone's SoC to drive the IoT.
Melanoma detection	A smartphone camera; the matching of suspicious image pattern with a library of images of cancerous skin; the app runs on the software platform in the smartphone's SoC to drive the IoT.
Remote surgery	Surgical robot systems and augmented reality sensors; robot arms, a master controller, and a feedback sensory system giving feedback to the user to ensure telepresence; real-time data connectivity and information management systems.

TABLE 6.2 Smartphone–Based Healthcare Apps.

Apps	Descriptions
Health Assistant	Keeps track of a wide range of health parameters such as body water and fat, weight, BP, body temperature, lipids, the glucose level, and various physical activities.
Healthy Children	Can search for pediatricians by location and request their advise for quick answers.
Google Fit	Tracks the user's walking, running, and cycling activities.
Calorie Counter	Keeps track of food consumed by the user as well as his or her weight and measurements, among others.
Water Your Body	Reminds the user to drink water every day and tracks his or her water-drinking habits.
Noom Walk	Serves as a pedometer to count the user's steps at all times.
Pedometer	Records the number of steps the user takes and displays related information such as the number of calories burned per a unit of time.
Period Calendar	Keeps track of the best periods, cycles, and ovulation dates and helps the user achieve or prevent pregnancy.
Period Tracker	Keeps track of periods and forecasts fertility.
Instant Heart Rate	Measures the heart rate by using the smartphone's built-in camera to sense changes of the color of the fingertip, which is directly related to the pulse.
Cardiax Mobile ECG	Serves as a companion app for Cardiax Window's full-scale, 12-channel personal computer (PC) ECG system.
ECG Self-Monitoring	Serves as an authomatic ECG device by registering ECG data based on the built-in "ECG self-check" software.
ElektorCardioscope	Displays ECG data through a wireless terminal.
Runtastic Heart Rate	Measures the heart rate on a real-time basis.
Heart Rate Monitor	Checks the heart rate on a real-time basis.
Cardiomobile	Monitors cardiac rehabilitation remotely on a real-time basis.
Blood Pressure (BP) Watch	Collects, tracks, analyzes, and shares BP data.
Finger Blood Pressure Prank	Measures BP based on the finger print.
OnTrack Diabetes	Tracks blood glucose and medication to help manage diabetes.
Finger Print Thermometer	Determines body temperature from the finger print.
Body Temperature	Keeps track of body temperature and identifies its severity.
Medisafe Meds & Pill Reminder	Reminds the user of medication times.

TABLE 6.2 *(Continued)*

Apps	Descriptions
Dosecast edication Reminder	Reminds the user of medication times, tracks the inventory, and maintains a log for drug management.
Rehabilitation Game	Serves as interactive game facilitating the auditory rehabilitation of patients with hearing loss.
iOximeter	Calculates the pulse rate and SpO_2.
Eye Care Plus	Tests and monitors vision.
SkinVision	Keeps track of the user's skin health and enables the early discovery of any skin disorder.
Asthma Tracker and Log	Keeps track of the patient's asthma.

The healthcare equipment and its utilizations are expected to deal with important personal data such as private health data. For the purpose, such smart devices have to be linked with the global information network that allow the user to access the network at anytime, anyplace, and any location. So, the healthcare platform also concentrates on strikers.

In order to fully adopt IoT in the healthcare field, it is important to identify and analyze various features of IoT security and privacy, containing safety necessity, weaknesses, threat models, and remedies from a healthcare perspective (Figure 6.6).

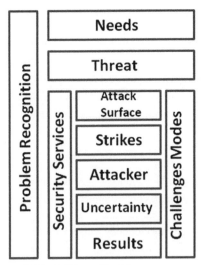

FIGURE 6.6 Security model for IoT-based healthcare.

1. Security necessities

Security necessity for IoT-based healthcare solutions can be understood by the standard communications schemes. Here, the followings are the some security-related requirements:

i) Private or secrete
Privacy ensures the restriction of medical report to unwanted users. In addition, confidential messages protest to reveal their content.

ii) Nobility
Nobility ensures that the available medical data are not being transmitted by an adverse transit. Moreover, the nobility of the stored data and content should not be compromised.

iii) Verification
Verification section should ensure the identity of sender who will be responsible for communicating.

iv) Availability
Availability ensures that selected parties, those were authorized only, will get the IoT healthcare service on priority basis either the entity will receive local or global service or in the case of denial-of-service condition.

v) Data freshness
Data freshness section ensures that the fresh messages are in the queue not old messages/information because IoT healthcare network concentrate on time-varying measurements.

vi) Nonrepudiation
Nonrepudiation refers to the node that had sent the information/message that must not deny for the case sent earlier.

vii) Authorization
This section ensures that only assigned nodes can approach the network services.

2. Security challenges

IoT security requirements were not ensured by traditional security methods; hence novel countermeasures are needed to address new challenges posed by the IoT. Various challenges for secure IoT healthcare services include the following parameters:

i) Memory limitations

Maximum IoT healthcare devices have very low on-device memory. Normally, these types of healthcare devices start with an operating system, application binary, and a system software. Hence, the inbuilt memory of healthcare devices cannot be sufficient to execute the complicated security protocols and store the very large information.

ii) Scalability

We know that day by day the quantity of IoT devices has been increased. Due to this reason, global information system is connected with the maximum IoT devices.

iii) IoT development boards

The development of suitable IoT boards for healthcare is also a security challenge. Various IoT boards are available in market such as Arduino Yun, Intel Galileo, Microduino, BeagleBone, and Intel Edison. Every IoT board has separate security challenges as per the operation requirements. Normally, Intel Edison IoT board is more used as compared to other IoT development boards. Intel Edison is a computer module. It enables creation of prototypes and fast development of prototype projects and rapidly produces IoT and wearable computing devices. It enables seamless device Internetworking and device-to-cloud communication. It includes the foundational tools. The tools collect the information, store and process data in the cloud, and process rules on the data stream. It generates triggers and alerts based on advanced analytics.

iv) Mobility

The feature of mobility is also very important for any medical-IoT network. This facility is mainly responsible for connecting the discontented patient environment. Some IoT healthcare networks have the ability to support the movement of patient to anywhere at anytime.

v) A multiprotocol network

A proprietary network protocol is required for the communication between one health device and another network in the local area network.

6.3.3 IoT HEALTHCARE TECHNOLOGIES

There are many capable technologies for IoT-based healthcare solutions; and therefore, it is a separate cult to create a clear list. In this regard, the main discussions on various key technologies that have the potential to fundamentally IoT-based healthcare services are as follows:

i. Cloud computing

Various researches have been carried out in recent years about cloud benefits for the applications of healthcare. These benefits have come from three primary services, which can be provided by cloud technologies in healthcare environments:

- Software as a Service—this service is used by healthcare providers and through this, the providers can work on health data and able to perform related tasks.
- Platform as a Service—this service helps in managing database, networking, virtualization, etc.
- Infrastructure as a Service—this service provides physical infrastructure for storage, servers, and many more.

These services can be used to obtain various types of tasks. Integration of cloud computing and IoT-based healthcare technologies should give facilities with universal access to shared resources, provide services on request to the structure, and perform operations to meet various requirements.

ii. Grid computing

An insufficient computational potential of medical sensor nodes can be addressed by starting grid computing for ubiquitous healthcare networks. It can be seen as the backbone of more accurate cluster and cloud computing.

iii. Big data

Big data may take large amounts of necessary health data generated from various medical sensors and give tools to increase the efficiency of relevant health diagnostics and monitoring methods and stages.

The main objection in big data management occurs in modeling a new system that can handle the attributes of a specific big data set. In healthcare, each specialty is important for 5 Vs, because the data taken at regular intervals from the patient's name, age, and gender to various important values need to be stored for different systems. Regularly measured data will create significant velocity and rapidly increase the amount of total data.

iv. Networks

From long-distance communication to networks to various networks, long-distance communication of the physical infrastructure of IoT-based healthcare is the part. A WSN in that environment is generally self-configuring, self-organizing, and self-discovering.

v. Ambient intelligence

Because the end users, customers, and clients are in the work of a healthcare person, the application of ambient intelligence is very important. With the help of ambient intelligence, we can easily learn about the human behavior and any necessary action is optimized by a recognized event. By the joining of human–computer interaction and integration of autonomous control technologies into ambient intelligence can further increase the capacity of IoT-assisted health services.

vi. Augmented reality

Augmented reality has an important position in healthcare industries as the part of IoT. Augmented reality is useful for surgery and remote observation and among others.

vii. Wearables

Patient commitment and population health reforms can be made accessible by wearing embraceable medical devices as places. These devices are very helpful to find the information about physical activities of patients. There are three major advantages:

- Information-connected information
- Healthcare target–oriented healthcare society
- Gamification

6.3.4 HEALTHCARE CHALLENGES OF IoT

Various models are designed and implemented on IoT-based healthcare services by various researchers to solve many problems related with those services. Despite the promise of what IoT can achieve in healthcare, the challenges are being faced. If these challenges were not resolved quickly, they could put IoT at a risk of failure.

Through intent and design, IoT equipment collect and transmit real-time data. The infrastructure needed to obtain and process this message must be designed and developed for scale. This means that acquisition, processing, and storage of data from millions of IoT devices in real time are evaluated by implementing analytics to gain insights from this data. Regrettably, most providers know how to access the data and how much lack of infrastructure is present.

However, healthcare data lack due to problems occurs in security and standards. This has always become a concern matter for IT professionals. Some challenges are discussed next:

i. Data privacy and security

The data privacy and security are the main challenges for any health IoT system. IoT system captures and transmits data in real time. Maximum IoT devices have less data protocols and standards. The security challenge of the data stored by different sensors is the challenge. IoT will allow healthcare providers to treat or observe the patient by focusing on relevant issues. Patient data can be misused to make fake IDs for cybercriminals to buy drugs or any other illegal activities.

ii. Accuracy and data overload

Communication model uses different protocols and standards, which becomes obstacle in the aggregation of data. These problems overcome by IoT. IoT devices are utilized to enhance vital insights. The stakeholders also are working on manual as logged work, which helps IoT devices to maintain the accuracy and data overload.

iii. Cost

The cost consideration is also a main challenge for any system. The main target of researchers is to reduce the cost of IoT-based healthcare services.

Cost factor is very concentrated point; while implementing a new setup, the researchers continuously work on the reduced cost of IoT-based healthcare service. The increasing medical cost becomes the worrying sign for esteemed country. While implementing the IoT, the stakeholders' main concentration is on optimization of cost-effectiveness so that the technology is reachable in every small and esteemed company.

iv. The business model

Finding the right and suitable business model is also a main challenge for any IoT healthcare system. An IoT healthcare business model added many requirements like operational policies and processes and transformed organizational models and distributed target customers.

v. Mobility

The feature of mobility is also very important for any medical-IoT network. This facility is mainly responsible for connecting the discontented patient environment. Any IoT healthcare network has the capability to support the movement of patient to anywhere at anytime.

6.3.5 IoT HEALTHCARE BENEFITS

i) Simultaneous monitoring and reporting

Real-time monitoring is very useful in the case of emergency like diabetes, heart attacks, and asthma attacks. In the real-time monitoring system, medical devices are connected with smartphone apps to provide the required necessary data, which is useful to any doctor and hospitals for doing the best treatment.

The IoT devices collect and transmit the health data like blood sugar levels, ECG, blood pressure, and weight. The role of the IoT device in healthcare is to collect, store the data at cloud, and share this data with doctor and insurance company or any external consultant at anytime, anyplace, or anywhere.

Apart from monitoring, there are various other important regions where IoT devices are very important in hospitals. For tracking the real-time location of instruments at hospitals, all used IoT devices are tagged with sensors. The most important concern for patients is the spread of infections.

ii) Good patient experience

A good healthcare system generates better environment as per the requirement of patients. For better patient experience, healthcare system must have the dedicated procedures, improved diagnosis accuracy, and enhanced treatment options.

iii) Home care

Home care service has been benefited for those patients who are not able to visit the hospital frequently. Here, monitoring of patient can be done by allowing M2M process with regard to patient's comfort. The collected data are shared with the hospital by cloud storage. Therefore, the IoT makes a revolution in the healthcare sector.

iv) Data assortment and analysis

At the cloud part, it is mandatory to free the space that is used by raw data. The IoT devices collect the report and analysis data with the help of providers. The providers acquire data from various devices and analyze by getting access to final report with graph.

v) Tracking and alerts

In severely debilitating conditions, on-time alert and tracking become critical. In that case, IoT allows the devices to collect and transfer the data to doctors with real-time tracking. This real-time tracking can be possible by dropping alert message to people via mobile applications.

Report and alert give strong opinion about the patient, despite the location and time. It also helps in knowing well-informed and timely treatment.

6.3.6 IoT HEALTHCARE DEVICES

A wide variety of smart instruments in healthcare that monitor the patient's state and well-being can be grouped in various ways with their different purposes. The relative graph of IoT-connected devices in worldwide from 2015 to 2025 is shown in Figure 6.7.[14]

i) Patient and staff behavior tracking appliances

The breathing rate, body temperature, body posture, and heart rate are measured by some tracking devices. These measuring devices have fall detection feature.

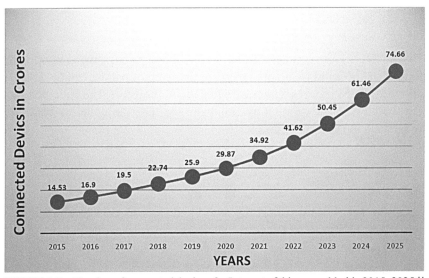

FIGURE 6.7 Number of connected devices for Internet of things worldwide 2015–2025.[14]

ii) Charting

IoT introduces new feature in healthcare system, that is, Audemix, which reduces doctor's manual work during the examination of patient. Audemix works on voice command and stores the patient information. This saves doctor's time and that patient data could be accessed for review.

6.4 CONCLUSION

This chapter gives a comprehensive study to understand IoT technologies, applications, and smart industrial management trends in IoT-based medical and healthcare solutions. Besides that, this chapter has discussed all the possible visions, concepts, framework, benefits, utility, challenges, and limitations of IoT healthcare utilizations. Smart healthcare can help scale down issues of medical errors.

The IoT in healthcare has some challenges but smart technologies have a confident impact on delivering beneficial data and supporting patient care. The e-health system must be able to protect the information privacy and security. The IoT can much better satisfy the requirements of healthcare system by monitoring all information regarding the healthcare, medical equipment. It is also helpful to solve the problem in medical platform construction, production safety, and service levels of medical services. Based on our analysis of IoT in healthcare, we identified various application prospects and scope of IoT in the improvement of services of patients. In the coming days, a much smarter and interflowing medical management will become trend, which will prosper people at large.

KEYWORDS

- **Internet of things**
- **healthcare**
- **networks**
- **security**
- **authentication**
- **technologies**

REFERENCES

1. Niewolny, D. *How the Internet of Things Is Revolutionizing Healthcare*; Freescale Semiconductors, 18 Oct 2013.
2. Gope, P.; Hwang, T. BSN-Care: A Secure IoT-Based Modern Healthcare System Using Body Sensor Network. *IEEE Sens. J.* **2016,** *16* (5), 1368–1376.
3. Zhu, N.; et al. Bridging E-Health and the Internet of Things: The SPHERE Project. *IEEE Intell. Syst.* **2015,** *30* (4), 39–46.
4. Chang, S.-H.; Chiang, R.-D.; Wu, S.-J.; Chang, W.-T. A Context-Aware, Interactive M-Health System for Diabetics. *IT Prof.* **2016,** *18* (3), 14–22.
5. Pasluosta, C. F.; Gassner, H.; Winkler, J.; Klucken, J.; Eskofier, B. M. An Emerging Era in the Management of Parkinson's Disease: Wearable Technologies and the Internet of Things. *IEEE J. Biomed. Health Inf.* **2015,** *19* (6), 1873–1881.
6. Fan, Y. J.; Yin, Y. H.; Xu, L. D.; Zeng, Y.; Wu, F. IoT-Based Smart Rehabilitation System. *IEEE Trans. Ind. Inf.* **2014,** *10* (2), 1568–1577.

7. Vasanth, K.; Sbert, J. Creating Solutions for Health through Technology Innovation. *Texas Instru.* [Online]. http://www.ti.com/lit/wp/sszy006/sszy006.pdf (accessed Dec 7, 2014).
8. Istepanian, R. S. H.; Hu, S.; Philip, N. Y.; Sungoor, A. The Potential of Internet of M-Health Things "m-IoT" for Non-Invasive Glucose Level Sensing. In *Proceedings of the IEEE Annual International Conference Engineering in Medicine and Biology Society (EMBC)*, Aug/Sept 2011; pp 5264–5266.
9. Luo, J.; Chen, Y.; Tang, K.; Luo, J. Remote Monitoring Information System and Its Applications Based on the Internet of Things. In *IEEE Transactions Institute of Information on Photonic & Optic Communications, Beijing University of Posts & Telecommunications*, Beijing, China, Dec 2009; p 482.
10. Varkey, J. P.; Pompili, D.; Walls, T. Human Motion Recognition Using a Wireless Sensor-Based Wearable System. *Pers. Ubiquitous Comput.* **2011,** 1–14.
11. Jara, A. J.; Belchi, F. J.; Alcolea, A. F.; Santa, J.; Zamora-Izquierdo, M. A.; Gomez-Skarmeta, A. F. A Pharmaceutical Intelligent Information System to Detect Allergies and Adverse Drugs Reactions Based on Internet of Things. In *IEEE Transactions of PERCOM2010*, Mannheim, Mar. 2010; p 809.
12. Chen, M.; Gonzalez, S.; Vasilakos, A.; Cao, H.; Leung, V. C. Body Area Networks: A Survey. *Mob. Netw. Appl.* **2011,** *16* (2), 171.
13. https://medium.com/datadriveninvestor/4-stages-of-iot-architecture-explained-in-simple-words-b2ea8b4f777f.
14. Alam Tanweer, "A Reliable Communication Framework and Its Use in Internet of Things (IoT)," IJSRCSEIT, May-June'18, Volume 3, Issue 5, ISSN : 2456-3307, PP-450-456.
15. Liu, M.-L.; Tao, L,; Yan, Z. Internet of Things-Based Electrocardiogram Monitoring System. Chinese Patent 102 764 118 A, Nov 7, 2012.
16. Puustjarvi, J.; Puustjarvi, L. Automating Remote Monitoring and Information Therapy: An Opportunity to Practice Telemedicine in Developing Countries. In *Proceedings of the IST-Africa Conference*, May 2011; pp 1–9.
17. Guan, Z. J. Internet-of-Things Human Body Data Blood Pressure Collecting and Transmitting Device. Chinese Patent 202 821 362 U, Mar 27, 2013.
18. Xin, T. J.; Min, B.; Jie, J. Carry-On Blood Pressure/Pulse Rate/Blood Oxygen Monitoring Location Intelligent Terminal Based on Internet of Things. Chinese Patent 202 875 315 U, Apr 17, 2013.
19. Ruiz, M. N.; García, J. M.; Fernández, B. M. Body Temperature and Its Importance as a Vital Constant. *Rev. Enferm.* **2009,** *32* (9), 44–52.
20. Jian, Z.; Zhanli, W.; Zhuang, M. Temperature Measurement System and Method Based on Home Gateway. Chinese Patent 102 811 185 A, Dec 5, 2012.
21. Khattak, H. A.; Ruta, M.; Di Sciascio, E. CoAP-Based Healthcare Sensor Networks: A Survey. In *Proceedings of the 11th International Bhurban Conference on Applied Science Technology (IBCAST)*, Jan 2014; pp 499–503.
22. Larson, E. C.; Goel, M.; Boriello, G.; Heltshe, S.; Rosenfeld, M.; Patel, S. N. Spiro Smart: Using a Microphone to Measure Lung Function on a Mobile Phone. In *Proceedings of the ACM International Conference on Ubiquitous Computing*, Sept 2012, pp 280–289.
23. Larson, E. C.; Lee, T.; Liu, S.; Rosenfeld, M.; Patel, S. N. Accurate and Privacy Preserving Cough Sensing Using a Low-Cost Microphone. In *Proceedings of the ACM International Conference on Ubiquitous Computing*, Sept 2011; pp 375–384.

24. Kolici, V.; Spaho, E.; Matsuo, K.; Caballe, S.; Barolli, L.; Xhafa, F. Implementation of a Medical Support System Considering P2P and IoT Technologies. In *Proceedings of the 8th International Conference on Complex, Intelligence Software Intensive Systems (CISIS)*, Jul 2014; pp 101–106.
25. Vermesan, O.; Friess, P. Internet of Things Strategic Research and Innovation Agenda. In *Internet of Things – Converging Technologies for Smart Environment and Integrated Ecosystems*; River Publishers, 2013; p 54.
26. Pang, Z. Technologies and Architectures of the Internet-of-Things (IoT) for Health and Well-being. Doctoral Thesis, KTH–Royal Institute of Technology Stockholm, Sweden, January 2013.
27. Xu, B.; Xu, L. D.; Cai, H.; Xie, C.; Hu, J.; Bu, F. Ubiquitous Data Accessing Method in IoT-Based Information System for Emergency Medical Services. *IEEE Trans. Ind. Inf.* **2014**, *10* (2), 1578–1586.
28. Churcher, G.; Bilchev, G.; Foley, J.; Gedge, R.; Mizutani, T. Experiences Applying Sensor Web Enablement to a Practical Telecare Application. In *Wireless Pervasive Computing, 2008. ISWPC 2008. 3rd International Symposium on*, May 2008; pp 138–142.
29. Pang, G.; Ma, C. A Neo-Reflective Wrist Pulse Oximeter. *IEEE Access* **2014**, 2, pp 1562–1567.
30. Internet of Things Needs Government Support. [Online]. http://www.informationweek.com/government/leadership/internet-of-things-needs-government-support/a/d-id/1316455 (accessed Dec 27, 2014).
31. Building Foundations for e-Health: Republic of Korea. [Online]. http://www.who.int/goe/data/country_report/kor.pdf (accessed Dec 27, 2014).
32. Mobile Health (m-Health) for Tobacco Control. [Online]. http://www.who.int/tobacco/mhealth/en (accessed Dec 27, 2014).
33. Directory of e-Health Policies. [Online]. http://www.who.int/goe/policies/en (accessed Dec 27, 2014).
34. A Family of Products to Help You Stay Healthy. [Online]. http://www.ihealthlabs.com (accessed Jan 10, 2015).
35. A Heart Rate Tracker You Can Count on. [Online]. http://www.mybasis.com (accessed Jan 10, 2015).
36. W/Me Wearable Wellness Monitor and Coach. [Online]. http://appleinsider.com/articles/13/12/18/review-wme-wearable-wellness-monitor-and-coach (accessed Jan 10, 2015).
37. Lijun, Z. Multi-Parameter Medical Acquisition Detector Based on Internet of Things. Chinese Patent 202 960 774 U; Jun 5, 2013.
38. Yue-Hong, Y.; Wu, F.; Jie, F. Y.; Jian, L.; Chao, X.; Yi, Z. Remote Medical Rehabilitation System in Smart City. Chinese Patent 103 488 880 A; Jan 1, 2014.
39. Liang, S.; Zilong, Y.; Hai, S.; Trinidad, M. Childhood Autism Language Training System and Internet-of-Things-based Centralized Training Center. Chinese Patent 102 184 661 A; Sept 14, 2011.
40. Pang, Z.; Tian, J.; Chen, Q. Intelligent Packaging and Intelligent Medicine Box for Medication Management Towards the Internet-of-Things. In *Proceedings of the 16th International Conference on Advance Communication Technology (ICACT)*, Feb 2014; pp 352–360.

41. Zhang, X. M.; Zhang, N. An Open, Secure and Exible Platform Based on Internet of Things and Cloud Computing for Ambient Aiding Living and Telemedicine. In *Proceedings of the International Conference on Computer Management (CAMAN)*, May 2011; pp 1–4.
42. Shahamabadi, M. S.; Ali, B. B. M.; Varahram, P.; Jara, A. J. A Network Mobility Solution Based on 6LoWPAN Hospital Wireless Sensor Network (NEMO-HWSN). In *Proceedings of the 7th International Conference on Innovative Mobile and Internet Services in Ubiquitous Computing (IMIS)*, Jul 2013; pp 433–438.
43. Jara, A. J.; Alcolea, A. F.; Zamora, M. A.; Skarmeta, A. F. J.; Alsaedy, M. Drugs Interaction Checker Based on IoT. In *Proceedings of the Internet Things (IOT)*, Nov/Dec 2010; pp 1–8.
44. Wei, L.; Heng, Y.; Lin, W. Y. Things Based Wireless Data Transmission of Blood Glucose Measuring Instruments. Chinese Patent 202 154 684 U; Mar 7, 2012.
45. Sajid, A.; Abbas, H. Data Privacy in Cloud-Assisted Healthcare Systems: State of the Art and Future Challenges. *J. Med. Syst.* **2016**, *42*(250). https://doi.org/10.1007/s10916-015-0327-y.
46. Sawand, A.; Djahel, S.; Zhang, Z.; Abdesselam, F. N. Toward Energy-Efficient and Trustworthy eHealth Monitoring System. *China Commun.* **2015**, *2* (1), 46–65.
47. Saxena, D.; Ray Choudhary, V. Design and Verification of an NDN-Based Safety-Critical Application: A Case Study with Smart Healthcare. *IEEE Trans. Syst. Man Cybern.: Syst.* **2017**, 1–15.
48. Zeadally, S.; Jesus, T.; Zubair, B. Security Attacks and Solutions in Electronic Health (E-health) Systems. *J. Med. Syst.* **2016**, *42* (251), 263.
49. Yang, L.; Ge, Y.; Li, W.; Rao, W.; Shen, W. A Home Mobile Healthcare System for Wheelchair Users. In *Proceedings of the IEEE International Conference on Computer Supported Cooperation Work Design (CSCWD)*, May 2014; pp 609–614.
50. Dash, P. K. Electrocardiogram Monitoring. *Indian J. Anaesth.* **2002**, *46* (4), pp 251–260.

CHAPTER 7

ODONTOGENIC TUMORS: PREVALENCE AND DEMOGRAPHIC DISTRIBUTION THROUGH IoT

PRIYANKA DEBTA[1], SIBANI SARANGI[1], DEBABRATA SINGH[2*], ANURAG DANI[3], SOMALEE MAHAPATRA[4], and MITRABINDA KHUNTIA[2]

[1]*I. D. S., Siksha 'O' Anusandhan, Deemed to be University, Bhubaneswar, Odisha, India*

[2]*ITER, Department of CSE, Siksha 'O' Anusandhan, Deemed to be University, Bhubaneswar, Odisha, India*

[3]*Department of Prosthodontia, C. D. C. R. I., Rajnandgaon, Chhattisgarh, India*

[4]*Department of Pathology and Microbiology, Hitech Dental College & Hospitals, Bhubaneswar, Odisha, India*

[*]*Corresponding author. E-mail: debabratasingh@soa.ac.in*

ABSTRACT

Recent developments in the Internet of Things (IoT) technology have produced extensive opportunities and innovations in the healthcare field. IoT-enabled healthcare has been a research domain that focuses on "the utilization of IoT-enabled methods and technologies to offer high-quality health services, including faster and safer preventive care, lower overall cost, improved patient-centered practice, and enhanced sustainability." Specific attention in this domain has been directed to traditional IoT technological studies including sensing, networking and communication, data mining, and human–computer interaction and healthcare. Healthcare supervising administrators in the hospitals and other health center staffs have to confirm all through the enormous development of the wireless healthcare counseling equipments along with numerous electronics components have become to enormous significance in many nations throughout the world.

Modern advancements have been centralized on the above methods of particular wireless body area network and wearable node to encounter signals like body temperature, pulse rate, and blood pressure. Hence fore, wireless sensor network technology could be engaged in demanding settings to assemble patient vital parameters. The collected data are broadcasted wirelessly over the receiving station associated with a warehouse where the data are prepared hypothetically which contributes relevant to security as well as confidentiality about the patient data, in conjunction with the avoidance of illegal approach or use of patient data, in addition, to ensure reliable real-time patient monitoring. In this paper, secured healthcare supervising system adopting a fuzzy logic-based decision platform which helps in resolving the Odontogenic tumors with you and your friend or loved one is proposed. Thus, an aggregation of fuzzy logic as well as protected flexible model is made use of in order to identify the status of the health of the patient taking into account of the neural network which is trained continuously as well as it has the capability to modify itself along with the changes in the input for which the desired output is assigned.

7.1 INTRODUCTION

The Internet of Things (IoT) is a new milestone in the digital era whereby physical objects can communicate with each other and function without human dependency.[1] These objects are termed as smart devices and can be controlled by an app installed on your Smartphone's. The main reason they are called smart is due to their built-in sensors that actually collect data for further analysis and action. IoT can be applied to every sphere of our life where electronic objects are used which is embedded with a networking chip for enabling them with IoT that will help in remote access and regulation. The scope of IoT is wide and is rapidly becoming a part of our everyday life.

The paper comes up with the aims at the discrimination accuracy with the organizing the technology of artificial intelligence, for instance the neural networks as well as the fuzzy system in achieving healthcare supervising organizations following the implementation of the system to work as an effective healthcare model that determines the preferences as such determined by the collected health specifications from various sensor nodes.[2] Healthcare counseling will continue in order to record the patient's body parameters as well as to maintain stability as well as steady data by the doctors or the medical team for diagnosis. This path will resolve in helping the patients in greater extent especially when needed in case of medical emergencies like depression due to odontogenic tumors.

Medical diagnosis consumes a huge amount of hospital bills. Technology can move the routines of medical checks from hospital (hospital-centric) to the patient's home (home-centric).[3] So, the most important application of IoT is its use in healthcare. The full application of this paradigm in the healthcare area is a mutual hope because it allows medical centers to function more competently and the patients to obtain better treatments. IoT application development companies[3] have offered impressive IoT-based health monitoring systems and tools, wearables, and mobile healthcare apps that make use of real-time data to offer significant information to the users. Such devices allow tracking, monitoring, and management in order to improve the precision, speed, and planning. The beauty of IoT in healthcare and life science is personalized medicine. Some of the benefits of using IoT in healthcare system are as follows:

1. *Simultaneous reporting and monitoring:* Real-time monitoring via connected devices can save lives in event of a medical emergency like heart failure, diabetes, asthma attacks, etc. Connected devices can collect medical and other required health data and use the data connection of the smartphone to transfer collected information to a physician with real-time monitoring of the condition in place by means of a smart medical device connected to a smartphone app. The IoT device collects and transfers health data: blood pressure, oxygen, and blood sugar levels, weight, and ECGs.[4]
2. *Improved disease management:* IoT-enabled devices allow real-time monitoring of patients which means no data in relation to the condition of the patient are missed, for example, the heart rate, blood pressure, body temperature, etc.[5,6] This facilitates the proper diagnosis of the illness. The IoT devices are also interconnected which means that they can be programed to give the immediate assistance that is required. The IoT devices can be set up with a higher or lower value limit. It will automatically trigger another connected device that will help to stabilize the condition of the patients; in any case of the devices that register a higher or lower

value limit. Simultaneously, it will also trigger an alert to the app in the smartphone of the doctor or nurse or the caregivers that ensure the constant medical assistance that is required in intensive units in hospitals.

3. *Remote monitoring of health:* IoT-enabled smart devices allows for patients to be monitored remotely as well.[7] The smart devices will collect constant data even if the patient is not in the hospital such as the blood pressure and temperature wearable is a small smart device that can be worn on the wrist which will help to monitor the heartbeat, blood pressure, and the body temperature of the patient. The high and the low indicators can be set at particular levels which when reached will send out an alert to the app in the smartphone of the patient or caregiver and the patient can be given the required medical attention right away.

4. *Connected healthcare and virtual infrastructure:* The data collected by IoT-enabled devices are stored in the cloud which makes its storage and access easy for future reference or remote study.[8] As well as the data collected by the smart devices in real time and can be accessed from anywhere by the Internet which becomes possible to provide the healthcare remotely. This means that even if the specialist is not located near the patient, he can still get the required assistance as his condition can be monitored remotely and diagnosed accurately. IoT in healthcare enables interoperability, machine-to-machine communication, information exchange, and data movement that make healthcare service delivery effective. IoT-enabled devices can go a long way toward helping people in locations where there are no proper hospitals and staff. Remote access can allow doctors and nurses to monitor and diagnose illness to provide basic and vital healthcare that is required.

5. *Accurate data collection and its availability:* The constant automated monitoring of the patient allows for accurate data collection without the possibility of error which enhances the study of the patient's condition leading to proper diagnosis and precise treatment as well as this data can be stored for future reference.[9] In case, a doctor must refer to the case history of the patient by accessing it via the IoT cloud and have a better understanding of the patient's condition which is applicable in case of emergencies as well as when immediate assistance is required and there may

not be enough time to contact the family for post conditions and sensitivities. Access to the IoT data can provide the data immediately enhancing the medical attention that the patient requires. IoT devices also help the doctors in patient charting which otherwise would have taken hours to complete.
6. *Drug management:* IoT has introduced talking devices that will remind patients of the medication that they need to take which enhances the timely delivery of drugs especially to elderly people suffering from blood pressure, diabetes, Alzheimer etc.[10]
7. *Emergency:* Remote monitoring of the patients with the help of the IoT wearable has made it possible to keep a real time track of health conditions. Any indication that the patient will be requiring immediate medical attention will alert the hospital and the patient can be brought to the hospital in time to receive emergency medical care. This is definitely a life over as time is a huge factor in giving the right treatment to avoid complications and reduce risk.

7.1.1 ODONTOGENIC TUMORS

Odontogenic tumors are relatively rare, slow-growing cellular proliferation with a broad spectrum of biologic potentials, and behaviors.[11,13] Present predominantly in the jaw these tumors represent an array of lesions ranging from malignant and benign neoplasm to tumor like malformations (hamartomas).[12] Despite its generalized characteristic feature of development from odontogenic residues, that is, odontogenic epithelia and/or ectomesenchyme reflecting the same sequence as of normal odontogenesis, odontogenic tumor does not completely rule out its origin from a pre-existing developmental cyst.[11,12] In many cases, the histogenesis may be only inferred from its site and structure.[12]

Odontogenic tumors include classic biology compiled together to be collectively termed as tumor which implies a deformed or abnormal increase in the cellular mass.

7.2 PATHOGENESIS

Odontogenic tumors arising from odontogenic residues, that is, ectomesenchyme and odontogenic with hard tissues (variable amounts) formed generally in the same sequence as in normal tooth development.[11] These tumors mimic normal odontogenesis featuring varying inductive interactions between odontogenic epithelium and odontogenic ectomesenchyme.[14,15] So, the classification of odontogenic tumors is essentially based on interactions between odontogenic ectomesenchyme and epithelium. 1) Tumors of odontogenic epithelium, 2) Mixed odontogenic tumors, and 3) Tumors of odontogenic ectomesenchyme.

7.2.1 CLASSIFICATION

However, this classification is under constant renewal because of the dynamic equilibrium between new entities and some older entities achieved by addition of the former and removal of the later.

The following classification summarizes the slow progressive modification of odontogenic tumors from the first WHO Classification (in 19710) to its latest classification (in 2017).

7.2.2 WHO CLASSIFICATION [1971]

7.2.2.1 BENIGN ODONTOGENIC TUMOR

The complex interaction in the teeth is primitive ectomesenchymal and ectoderm tissues. Generally, human have two sets of teeth (permanent and deciduous), odontogenesis is a prolonged biologic process. Odontogenic tissues are present always in our bone or soft tissues of the jaw, even after Odontogenesis process.[30]

Benign odontogenic tumor can be classified as:

 i. Ameloblastoma
 ii. Calcifying epithelial odontogenic tumor
 iii. Ameloblastic fibroma
 iv. Adenomatoid odontogenic tumor
 v. Calcifying odontogenic cyst
 vi. Dentinoma
 vii. Ameloblastic fibro odontoma
 viii. Odonto ameloblastoma
 ix. Complex odontoma

x. Compound odontoma
xi. Fibroma
xii. Myxoma (myxofibroma)
xiii. Cementomas

Here, Cementomas is further classified as[31]

a) Benign cementoblastoma, b) Cementifying fibroma, c) Periapical cemental dysplasia, d) Gigantiform cementoma (familial multiple cementoma).

7.2.2.2 MALIGNANT ODONTOGENIC TUMORS

Odontogenic neoplasms derive from mesenchymal remnants and epithelial of the tooth germ which can be classified into benign and malignant tumors. The malignant odontogenic tumors or neoplasms are extremely challenging nowadays. Odontogenic malignancies tumors are extremely rare and complicated, which can be diagnosed by the biological behavior, diagnostic methods, reproducible standardized criteria, clinical management, and appropriate classification. Malignant odontogenic tumors can be classified as:

1. ODONTOGENIC CARCINOMAS
    a) Malignant ameloblastoma
    b) Primary intraosseous carcinoma
    c) Other carcinomas arising from odontogenic epithelium, including those arising from odontogenic cysts.

2. ODONTOGENIC SARCOMAS
    a) Ameloblastic fibrosarcoma
    b) Ameloblastic odontosarcoma

7.2.3 WHO CLASSIFICATION (1992)

7.2.3.1 BENIGN ODONTOGENIC TUMORS

1. Epithelial origin
    a) Ameloblastoma
    b) Squamous odontogenic tumor
    c) Calcifying epithelial odontogenic tumor
    d) Clear cell odontogenic tumor

2. Mixed origin
   a) Ameloblastic fibroma
   b) Ameloblastic fibrodentinoma
   c) Odontoameloblastoma
   d) Adenomatoid odontogenic tumor
   e) Calcifying odontogenic cyst
   f) Complex odontoma
   g) Compound odontoma
3. Mesenchymal Origin
   a) Odontogenic fibroma
   b) Myxoma
   c) Benign cementoblastoma

7.2.3.2 MALIGNANT ODONTOGENIC TUMORS

A) Odontogenic Carcinomas: Odontogenic carcinomas are the odontogenic counterparts and malignant epithelial to the 2005 WHO classification of odontogenic tumors.

Odontogenic Carcinomas can be classified as: a) Malignant ameloblastoma, b) Primary intraosseous Carcinoma, c) Malignant variants of other odontogenic epithelial tumors, d) Malignant changes in odontogenic cysts.

7.2.4 WHO CLASSIFICATION (2005)

7.2.4.1 BENIGN ODONTOGENIC TUMOR

1. Epithelial origin: Carcinoma refers to a malignant neoplasm of epithelial origin or cancer of the internal or external lining of the body, Sometimes also it can be seen in myofibroblasts during fibrosis in the lungs. It can be classified as:

    a) Ameloblastoma (solid multicystic type), b) Ameloblastoma (extraosseous/peripheral type), c) Ameloblastoma desmoplastic type, d) Ameloblastoma unicystic type, e) Squamous odontogenic tumor, f) Calcifying epithelial odontogenic tumor, g) Adenomatoid odontogenic tumor, and h) Keratocystic odontogenic tumor.

2. Mixed tumor
   a) Ameloblastic fibroma, b) Ameloblastic fibrodentinoma, c) Ameloblastic fibro-odontoma, d) Complex odontoma, e) Compound odontoma f) Odontoameloblastoma, g) Calcifying cystic odontogenic tumor, and h) Dentinogenic ghost cell tumor,
3. Mesenchymal origin
   a) Odontogenic fibroma, b) Odontogenic myxoma/Myxofibroma, and c) Cementoblastoma

7.2.4.2 MALIGNANT ODONTOGENIC TUMORS

1. Odontogenic carcinomas
   a) Malignant ameloblastoma/metastasizing ameloblastomas
   b) Ameloblastic carcinoma-primary type
   c) Ameloblastic carcinoma-secondary type, intraosseous
   d) Ameloblastic carcinoma-secondary type, peripheral
   e) Primary intraosseous scc-solid type
   f) Primary intraosseous scc derived from odontogenic cysts
   g) Clear cell odontogenic carcinoma
   h) Ghost cell odontogenic carcinoma
2. Odontogenic sarcomas
   a) Ameloblastic fibrosarcoma
   b) Ameloblastic fibrodentino and fibro odontosarcoma.

7.2.5 WHO CLASSIFICATION (2017)

7.2.5.1 BENIGN ODONTOGENIC TUMORS

1. Epithelial origin
   a) Ameloblastoma
      -Unicystic type
      -Extraosseous/peripheral type
      -Metastasizing ameloblastoma
   b) Squamous odontogenic tumor
   c) Calcifying epithelial odontogenic tumor
   d) Adenomatoid odontogenic tumor

2. Mixed origin
   a) Ameloblastic fibroma
   b) Primordial odontogenic tumor
   c) Complex odontoma
   d) Compound odontoma
   e) Dentinogenic ghost cell tumor
3. Mesenchymal origin
   a) Odontogenic fibroma
   b) Myxofibroma
   c) Cementoblastoma
   d) Cement-ossifying fibroma

7.2.5.2 MALIGNANT ODONTOGENIC TUMORS[19]

1. Odontogenic Carcinomas
   a) Ameloblastic carcinoma
   b) Primary intraosseous carcinoma
   c) Sclerosing odontogenic carcinoma
   d) Clear cell odontogenic carcinoma
   e) Ghost cell odontogenic carcinoma
2. Odontogenic carcinosarcomas
3. Odontogenic sarcomas

7.3 PREVELANCE OF ODONTOGENIC TUMORS IN INDIA

In India, the frequency of reported odontogenic tumors is quite less owing to the existing ethnical diversity based on caste, language, and geographic variations which is further catalyzed by scarce studies on the same.[16,18]

Following are few reported cases of odontogenic tumors reported from various parts of India. These cases have been further studied and analyzed on the basis of certain criteria and various inferences deduced out of this study helps us to understand odontogenic tumors in a better lucid manner and guiding the further research and study to a better confined way.

7.3.1 I-DEMOGRAPHIC DISTRIBUTION OF VARIOUS TYPES OF ODONTOGENIC TUMORS IN VARIOUS REGIONS ON BASIS OF AGE

7.3.1.1 AMELOBLASTOMA

Ameloblastoma has been reported to be one of the most commonly reported cases of odontogenic tumors. According to a retrospective study carried out in the state of Maharashtra by MS Ahire et al.[19] in the year 2018, on 250 samples of odontogenic tumors collected, 77 cases constituting approximately 30.8% turned out to be ameloblastoma. It showed its maximum frequency in the age group of 19–39 years, that is, 23 out of 77 cases (29.8%) in age group of 19–20 years, 14 out of 77 cases (18.18%) in age group of 21–30 years, 14 out of 77 cases (18.18%) in age group of 30–39 years.

Comparing the study with another study group conducted in the state of Andhra Pradesh at an institutional set up by Nalabolu GRK et al.[17] in the year 2017, it was found that out of 161 samples of identified odontogenic tumors reported in between the year 2002–2014, ameloblastoma was reportedly found in the age group of 11–50 years with a peak incidence in the age group of 21–30 years. Like the previous study in the state of Maharashtra, ameloblastoma also shows highest incidence among the south Indian population counting its number to 79 out of 161 cases, that is, 49.06%.

The above study can be compared to a retrospective study carried out in the state of Odisha by S Ramachandra et al.[18] in the year 2014 on the 76 samples collected over a period of 5 years, that is, from 2007 to 2012. Still bagging its highest frequency among very few reported odontogenic tumor cases, that is, 52 out of 76 cases (i.e., approx. 68.42%), ameloblastoma shows its peak incidence in the age group of 21–40 years (76.92%) followed by age above 50 years (17.30%) and least among age group of below 20 years (5.76%). This result shows contrast with the distribution of ameloblastoma among the south Indian population as the latter state shows more distribution of ameloblastoma among the population in the age group of 11–20 (i.e., 21.5%) than the former state which shows a minimal prevalence among the age group of 11–20 years (i.e., 5.76%).

7.3.2 ODONTOMA

Odontoma is the second most reported tumor among the samples of odontogenic tumor studied in various parts of India. Comparing the results of various studies in different population group showed the following results: Odontoma has approximately 19.2% in maharastra[19] distributed among wide array of age group, that is, 4 out of 250 (i.e., 1.6%) in 0–9 years, 18 out of 250 (7.2%) in 10–19 years, 10 out of 250 (4%) in 19–20 years, 7 out of 250 (2.8%) in 20–29 years, 3 out of 250 (1.2%) in 30–39 years, 3 out of 250 (1.2%) in 40–49 years, 2 out of 250 (0.8%) in 50–59, and 1 out of 250 (0.4%) in 90–99 years.

In south Indian states, according to the conducted retrospective study,[17] 10 samples showed positive findings for odontoma constituting 6.2% of the total odontogenic tumors. Unlike the study by MS Ahire et al.,[19] it shows its distribution to limited population, that is, equal predilection of 5 out of 10 cases (50%) in age group of below 20 years and the same frequency in the age group of 21–40 years, that is, (50%) with no evidence of odontoma in the age group above 50 years of age among the studied south Indian population as compared to the Maharashtra population[9] that showed approx. 6 out of 250 cases, that is, 2.4%.

However, the results of study by Nalabolu et al.,[17] somehow congruent the same pattern of distribution as the pattern analyzed among the Odisha population as per the study conducted by S. Ramachandra et al.,[18] out of 7.8% of reported odontomas, 66.66% of it, that is, (four out of six) showed the same incidence between 21 and 50 years of age and remaining 33.33% showed its presence around age below or up to 20 years. Like study of Nalabolu et al.,[17] there is no reported case of odontoma above 50 years of age.

7.3.3 ADENOMATOID ODONTOGENIC TUMOR

Adenomatoid odontogenic tumor ranks third among the frequency of odontogenic tumors. According to the study by MS Ahire et al.,[19] adenomatoid odontogenic tumor (AOT) has a frequency of 14%, that is, 35 out of 250 cases showing its maximum effect in younger age group of 10–19 years (68.5%) and a mean age of 18.89, followed by less frequent presence in the age group of 19–20 years, that is, 28.57% and rarely in age range of 20–29 years (2.8%).

However, the results for AOT in the study conducted in Andhra Pradesh and Odisha by Nalabolu et al.[17] and S Ramachandra et al.,[18] respectively, are quiet comparable showing a more or less similar pattern of distribution of AOT among the populations of Andhra Pradesh and Odisha.

The study[17] shows 9 out of 161 cases were AOT (5.59%) out of which 5 cases (55.55%) are found in age of 11–20 years, 2 cases (22.22%) in age of 21–30 years, and 1 case each (11.11%) in age group 31–40 years and 41–50 years.

The tudy[18] shows 6 out of 76 cases to be AOT (7.89%), with equal incidences in the age group of less than 20 years and between 21 and 50 years, that is, 50% in each age group.

The above study[19], hence, shows involvement of younger individuals mostly in the first and second decades of life with AOT in Maharashtra while in studies about Andhra Pradesh and Odisha[17,28]; the later, two states have high AOT predilection in the age group ranging from second to fifth decade of life.

7.4 AMELOBLASTIC FIBROMA

Ameloblastic fibroma is a rare type of odontogenic tumor that shows almost negligible prevalence in India.

In Maharashtra, ameloblastic fibroma is only found in 3 out of 250 odontogenic tumor samples (1.2%) in the first and second decades of life with the frequency of 33.33 and 66.66%, respectively.[29]

The study in Odisha[28], however, shows 5 out of 76 cases (6.5%) with ameloblastic fibroma. This rare frequency is found in among sample population in the age group of 21–50 years (three of five) and less than 20 years (two of five).

Andhra Pradesh has almost no reported cases of AOT among its study population except one case (0.62%) in the third decade of life.

7.5 CALCIFYING EPITHELIAL ODONTOGENIC TUMORS

Like Ameloblastic fibroma, Calcifying Epithelial Odontogenic Tumors (CEOT) has also less prevalence in Indian population.

In Maharashtra,[19] 4 out of 250 cases were diagnosed with calcifying epithelial odontogenic tumor (1.6%) which showed 1 case in between age of 10 and 19 years, 2 cases in age of 19–20 years and 1 case in age of 20–29 years.

Similar result is shared by the study population of Andhra Pradesh[17], with a mere frequency of 1.8% of CEOT out of 161 cases. One case is found in age group of 31–40 years and two cases are found in age of 41–50 years.

Odisha, however, shows higher prevalence of CEOT as compared to the states of Andhra Pradesh and Maharashtra.[18] This shows 3.95% of odontogenic tumor cases to be CEOT out of which two are found in the age range of 21–50 years and rarely one case above 50 years of age.

7.6 ODONTOGENIC MYXOMA

This odontogenic tumor shows equal prevalence in all the study populations analyzed across different parts of India.[17–19] They show 4 out of 161 cases (2.5%) in Andhra Pradesh,[7] 2 out of 76 cases in Odisha (2.63%)[8] and 6 out of 250 cases (2.4%) in Maharashtra.[19] In Andhra Pradesh and Maharashtra, they are found in the second and third decade of life[17,19], while in Odisha they are exclusively analyzed in the age range from third to fifth decade of life.

7.7 SQUAMOUS ODONTOGENIC TUMOR

Least reported odontogenic tumor, squamous odontogenic tumor was reported in very less frequency among the study population of Andhra Pradesh and Maharashtra[7,9] reported one and two cases in the fourth and first and second decade of life.[17,19] There is no such evidence of squamous odontogenic tumor in Odisha.[18]

7.7.1 DEMOGRAPHIC DISTRIBUTION OF VARIOUS ODONTOGENIC TUMORS ACCORDING TO GENDER AND ANATOMICAL SITE

7.7.1.1 AMELOBLASTOMA

  i) GENDER—Along with age predilection, ameloblastoma also shows gender predilection. In the study population of Odisha,[18] out of 52 cases of ameloblastoma (68.42%) 24 (46.15%) cases are found among males and 28 (53.84%) are found in females indicating female predilection. In Maharashtra, out of 77 (30.8%) cases of ameloblastoma, male count is 56 and female count is 21.[21] The further variants of ameloblastoma even show male predilection, that is, out of 46 (18.4%) cases of unicystic ameloblastoma, 26 cases are reported in males and 20 cases are reported in females. Similarly, peripheral ameloblastoma rarely reported to be one case that is found in male. In Andhra Pradesh study population,[17] out of 79 reported cases of ameloblastoma, majority of the cases are found in males, that is, 55 (69.62%) and 24 cases were found in females, that is, 30.39%. So, from the above comparison of ameloblastoma distribution on gender basis shows that the tumor shows slight female predilection in Odisha[8] which is in contrast to the states of Maharashtra and Andhra Pradesh[17,19] as the latter two states show male predilection.

ii) ANATOMICAL SITE OF DISTRIBUTION—Ameloblastoma is seen mostly habituating the mandible[4]; predominantly in the posterior aspects[4] shows: Posterior mandible (molar area-66%, premolar area-11%), Posterior maxilla (molar area-6%, premolar area-1%), Anterior mandible-10%, and anterior maxilla-6%.

In the study population of Odisha,[18] more prevalence of ameloblastoma was found in mandibular posterior aspect. In Andhra Pradesh[17], the results concordance with results of Odisha,[8] that is,

AMELOBLASTOMA

a) Anterior Maxilla-7 a) Anterior Mandible-14
b) Posterior Maxilla-9 b) Posterior mandible-49

In Maharashtra,[9] the results were analyzed in detail which was as follows;

AMELOBLASTOMA

a) Anterior Maxilla-3 a) Anterior Mandible-13
b) Posterior Maxilla-4 b) Posterior Mandible-46

UNICYSTIC AMELOBLASTOMA

a) Anterior maxilla-3 a) Anterior mandible-10
b) Posterior maxilla-1 b) Posterior Mandible-27

7.7.2 PERIPHERAL AMELOBLASTOMA

Comparing the results of the mentioned studies[17–19]; it reveals that ameloblastoma is not only the most dominant odontogenic tumor, but also one of the odontogenic tumors that habituates in the posterior aspect of mandible.

a) Anterior maxilla-0
b) Posterior maxilla-0

a) Anterior mandible-1
b) Posterior mandible-0

7.7.3 ODONTOMA

1. GENDER—In all the studies,[27–29] odontoma shows male predilection, that is, in Odisha, out of six reported cases of odontoma, four are found in males and two are found in females constituting 66.66 and 33.33%, respectively.[28] In Maharashtra, out of 48 cases of odontoma (19.2%), 24 cases are of males and 23 cases are of females.[9] In Andhra Pradesh, out of 10 cases of odontoma, 6 (60%) cases show male predilection whereas the remaining 4 (40%) cases show female predilection.[27] Thus, odontoma shows uniformity in its distribution on the basis of gender.[27–29]

2. ANATOMICAL SITE OF DISTRIBUTION—Unlike its uniformity in gender distribution, odontoma showed a heterogeneity in its anatomical site location. In Andhra Pradesh,[17] 10 cases were reported which showed the following gender distribution;

   a) Anterior Maxilla-5
   b) Posterior Maxilla-1

   a) Anterior Mandible-2
   b) Posterior Mandible-2

   In Maharashtra,[19] out of 40 cases with evidence of odontomas, the following gender distribution was found:

   a) Anterior maxilla-18
   b) Posterior maxilla-4

   a) Anterior mandible-3
   b) Posterior mandible-15

   In Odisha,[8] odontomas are predominantly found in the posterior mandible followed by anterior mandible. In rarest cases of odontomas, they are detected in anterior maxilla. Hence, the comparison of studies shows predominance of tumor in the maxilla (anterior in particular)[17,19] unlike the study[18] which shows mandibular dominance (posterior in particular).

7.7.4 ADENOMATOID ODONTOGENIC TUMOR

1. GENDER—the results for the study of distribution of AOT read as follows: in Odisha,[18] out of six reported cases of AOT, it has equal gender predilection of three and three in males and females, respectively. In Andhra Pradesh,[17] out of nine reported cases of AOT, six are found positive in males showing male predilection. In Maharashtra,[19] out of 35 cases of AOT, 19 are found in female patients and 16 are found in male patients showing female predilection. So, the comparison shows that AOT shows heterogeneity in all the study groups analyzed across different parts of India. In southern states, it has male predilection,[17] In western states it has female predilection[9] while in eastern states it has equal predilection.[8]
2. ANATOMICAL SITE OF DISTRIBUTION of the AOT Follows the following distribution pattern: in Odisha, the adenomatoid odontogenic tumor is found predominantly in the posterior aspects of mandible.[18] In Andhra Pradesh, AOT is found in the following sites at the following frequencies[17]: a) Anterior maxilla-5, b) Anterior mandible-2, c) Posterior Maxilla-1, d) Posterior mandible-1. In Maharashtra, AOT is found as[19];-

   a) Anterior maxilla-19   a) Anterior mandible-10
   b) Posterior maxilla-0   b) Posterior mandible-4

   So, the AOT shows its pre-dominance mostly in the maxilla (anterior to be particular) in Maharashtra and Andhra Pradesh[19,17] which differs from its distribution among the Odisha study population,[18] that is, posterior mandible.

7.7.5 AMELOBLASTIC FIBROMA

1. GENDER—In Odisha, ameloblastic fibroma has slight male predilection for being found among three out of five cases.[8] In Andhra Pradesh, ameloblastic fibroma is found rarely among the study population with only one reported case in male patient.[17] In Maharashtra, ameloblastic fibroma has female predilection with two out of three reported cases of ameloblastic fibroma.[9] So, studies[18,19] shows male predilection while study[26] shows female predilection.

ii) ANATOMICAL SITE OF DISTRIBUTION—Following are the results of ameloblastic fibroma on the basis of anatomical sites of distribution. In Odisha, it is predominantly found in the mandible (particularly posterior).[18] In Andhra Pradesh, it is rarely found and may be confined to anterior mandible.[7] In Maharashtra, it is found as:

a) Anterior maxilla-0   a) Anterior mandible-0
b) Posterior maxilla-1   b) Posterior mandible-2

so, the study shows mostly mandibular predilection.[27–29]

7.7.6 ODONTOGENIC MYXOMA

i) GENDER—The following are the results of odontogenic myxoma study: In Odisha, it is found in females only as per the analysis of the result deduced from the study population,[28] that is, two out of two cases.

In Andhra Pradesh, it shows similar pattern of female predilection, that is, three out of four reported cases.[27]

In Maharashtra, it shows female predilection with four out of six cases reported among females.[29]

So, the comparison of the results deduced from the above three studies carried out in different parts of India,[27–29] it is concluded that odontogenic myxoma shows homogeneity in its gender basis of distribution.

ii) ANATOMICAL SITE OF DISTRIBUTION—The following are the results of distribution: In Odisha, odontogenic myxoma is found predominantly in mandible than maxilla, that is, four out of six cases in mandible.[28] In Andhra Pradesh, odontogenic myxoma is found only in mandible as per the study analysis[27], that is, four out of four cases with further predominance in anterior mandible, that is, (three out of four) and in posterior mandible (one of four).[27] In Maharashtra, odontogenic myxoma is found as follows:- a) Anterior maxilla-1, b) Anterior mandible-1, c) Posterior maxilla-1, and d) Posterior mandible-3.

Hence, the above study reveals that like its gender predilection, odontogenic myxoma exhibits similar homogeneity in its pattern of distribution in various anatomical site, that is, mandible.[14,22]

However, there may be a negligible variation in its anterior-posterior distribution.[17,19]

7.8 CALCIFYING EPITHELIAL ODONTOGENIC TUMOR

i) GENDER—The following results are observed: In Maharashtra, it has male predilection, that is, (three out of four) cases were detected in males.[19] In Andhra Pradesh, it has similar male predilection, that is, (two out of three) cases are found in males and one in females.[17] In Odisha, it shows female predilection, that is, two out of three cases are reported in female patients.[18] Hence, Odisha stands out to be different in its gender predilection in comparison to the other two states as the former shows female predilection whereas the alter two states show male predilection.[17-19]

ii) ANATOMICAL SITE OF DISTRIBUTION—The following pattern is as follows:- In Odisha, this tumor is found only in posterior aspects of mandible .[18] In Andhra Pradesh, this tumor is also found in posterior mandible only.[17] In Maharashtra, this tumor is found at following sites:

a) Anterior maxilla-0   a) Anterior mandible-1
b) Posterior maxilla-2 b) Posterior mandible-1

So, comparing the above results we deduce that study of the south Indian states and eastern states[7,8] shows similar site prevalence in contrast to the western state[9] which shows equal site predilection.

7.9 SQUAMOUS ODONTOGENIC TUMORS

i) GENDER—The following are few findings illustrating the relative frequency of this tumor on the basis of age. In Andhra Pradesh, only 2 cases out of 161 cases were found to be squamous odontogenic tumor[17] and it was found in 2 female samples only in Maharashtra, even the number was negligible, that is, 1 out of 250 cases which was found in a male patient.[19] There was no cases of squamous odontogenic tumor reported in the study population of Odisha.

ii) ANATOMICAL SITE OF DISTRIBUTION—The following is the result: In Andhra Pradesh, it was sited predominantly in mandible with equal predilection in the anterior and posterior aspect, that is, (one and one).[17]

In Maharashtra, it is rarely spotted in the anterior aspect of mandible.[19]

Till now, other countries like Sri Lanka, Iran, Nigerian, Mexico, Chinese, Brazil studies have done related to prevalence and demographic distribution of odontogenic tumors.[10–18] Here, we focus and did an overview of odontogenic tumor's prevalence in various parts of India.

7.10 CONCLUSION

So after a keen observation and lucid discussion about various categories of odontogenic tumors under multiple classifications, various criteria we may conclude that odontogenic tumors are quite pseudopodic in their prevalence, pattern, and pathogenicity. With the similar histogenesis, these tumors show difference in their distribution, gender predilection, and site of inoculation. Further limited information resources and literature forms, are a hindrance in a detailed study about the prevalence of odontogenic tumors in all the parts of India. So, we should focus on expanding the scope of study on odontogenic tumors and scrutinize its features in all the parts of India with an aim to expand its scope of study and to make its clinical identification much precise and specific.

KEYWORDS

- fuzzy logic
- confidentiality
- Internet of things
- healthcare field
- communication
- data mining

REFERENCES

1. Gubbi, J.; Buyya, R.; Marusic, S.; Palaniswami, M. Internet of Things (IoT): A Vision, Architectural Elements, and Future Directions. *Future Gen. Comput. Syst.* **2013**, *29* (7), 1645–1660.
2. Elhoseny, M.; Ramírez-González, G.; Abu-Elnasr, O. M.; Shawkat, S. A.; Arunkumar, N.; Farouk, A. Secure Medical Data Transmission Model for IoT-based Healthcare Systems. *IEEE Access* **2018**, *6*, 20596–20608.
3. Da Xu, L.; He, W.; Li, S. Internet of Things in Industries: A Survey. *IEEE Trans. Ind. Info.* **2014**, *10* (4), 2233–2243.
4. Mikusz, M.; Clinch, S.; Jones, R.; Harding, M.; Winstanley, C.; Davies, N. Repurposing Web Analytics to Support the IoT. *Computer* **2015**, *48* (9), 42–49.
5. Dimitrov, D. V. Medical Internet of Things and Big Data in Healthcare. *Healthcare Info. Res.* **2016**, *22* (3), 156–163.
6. Pasluosta, C. F.; Gassner, H.; Winkler, J.; Klucken, J.; Eskofier, B. M. An Emerging Era in the Management of Parkinson's Disease: Wearable Technologies and the Internet of Things. *IEEE J. Biomed. Health Info.* **2015**, *19* (6), 1873–1881.
7. Hossain, M. S.; Muhammad, G. Cloud-assisted Industrial Internet of Things (IIoT) –Enabled Framework for Health Monitoring. *Comput. Netw.* **2016**, *101*, 192–202.
8. Nastic, S.; Sehic, S.; Le, D-H.; Truong, H-L.; Dustdar, S. Provisioning Software-defined IoT Cloud Systems. In *2014 International Conference on Future Internet of Things and Cloud*; IEEE, 2014; pp 288–295.
9. Sun, Y.; Song, H.; Jara, A. J.; Bie, R. Internet of Things and Big Data Analytics for Smart and Connected Communities. *IEEE Access* **2016**, *4*, 766–773.
10. Zanjal, S. V.; Talmale, G. R. Medicine Reminder and Monitoring System for Secure Health Using IOT. *Procedia Comput. Sci.* **2016**, *78*, 471–476.
11. Marx, R. E.; Stern, D. *Oral and Maxillofacial Pathology: A Rationale for Diagnosis and Treatment*. Hanover Park: Quintessence Publishing Company, 2012, pp 667–720.
12. Sivapathasundaram, B. *Shafers Textbook of Oral Pathology. Cysts and Tumors of Adontogeic Origin*, 7th ed.; Elsevier Publisher, 2012; pp 275–301.
13. Bhasker, S. N. Synopsis of Oral Pathology. Odontogenic Tumors of Jaw, Nonodontogenic Tumors and Pseudotumors of Jaw, 7th ed.; CBS Publishers, 1990; pp 260–364.
14. Neville. Oral and Maxillofacial Pathology. Odontogenic Cysts and Tumors, 3rd ed.; Elsevier Publication, 2011; pp 701–731.
15. Wright, J. M.; Soluk, T. M. Odontogenic Tumors. Where Are We in 2017? *J. Istanb. Univ. Fac. Dent.* **2017**, *51* (3 Suppl 1), S10–S30.
16. Lanje, A. H.; Misurya, R.; Chaudhary, M.; Gawande, M.; Hande, A.; Shukla, C. Odontogenic Tumors in India-A Review. *Int. J. Prev. Clin. Dent. Res.* **2017**, *4* (3), 235–237.
17. Nalabolu, G. R.; Mohiddin, A.; Hiremath, S. K. S.; Manyam, R.; Bharath, T. S.; Raju, P. R. Epidemiological Study of Odontogenic Tumors: An Institutional experience. *J. Infect. Public Health* **2017**, *10* (3), 324–330.
18. Ramachandra, S.; Shekar, P. C.; Prasad, S.; Kumar, K. K.; Reddy, G. S.; Prakash, K. L.; Reddy, B. V. Prevalence of Odontogenic Cysts and Tumors: A Retrospective Clinico-Pathological Study of 204 Cases. *SRM J. Res. Dent. Sci.* **2014**, *5*, 170–173.

19. Ahire, M. S.; Tupkari, J. V.; Chettiankandy, T. J.; Thakur, A.; Agrawal, R. R. Odontogenic Tumors: A 35-year Retrospective Study of 250 Cases in an Indian (Maharashtra) Teaching Institute. *Indian J. Cancer* **2018**, *55*, 265–272.
20. Okada, H.; Yamamoto, H.; Tilakratne, W. M. Odontogenic Tumors in Sri Lanka: Analysis of 226 Cases. *J. Oral Maxillofac. Surg.* **2007**, *65*, 875–882.
21. Kowkabi, M.; Razavi, S. M.; Khosravi, N.; Navabe, A. A. Odontogenic Tumors in Iran Isfaha. A Study of 260 Cases. *Dent. Res. J.* **2012**, *9*, 725–729.
22. Sagahravanian, N.; Jafarzadeh, H.; Bashardoost, N.; Pahalavan, N.; Shirinbak, I. Odontogenic Tumors in an Iraninan Population. A 30 Year Evaluation. *J. Oral Sci.* **2010**, *52*, 391–396.
23. Oluseyi, F. A.; Akinola, L. L.; Wasik, L. A.; Mobolanle, O. O. Odontogenic Tumors in Nigerian Children & Adoloscents. A Retrospective Study of 92 Cases. *World J. Surg. Oncol.* **2004**, *27*, 39.
24. Ramos Gde, O.; Porto, J. C.; Vieira, D. S.; Siqueira, F. M.; Rivero, E. R. Odontogenic Tumors: A 14-year Retrospective Study in Santa Catarina, Brazil. *Braz. Oral Res.* **2014**, *28*, 33–38.
25. Lu, Y.; Xuan, M.; Takata, T.; Wang, C.; He, Z.; Zhou, Z. et al. Odontogenic Tumors. A Demographic Study of 759 Cases in a Chinese Population. *Oral Surg. Oral Med. Oral Pathol. Oral Radiol. Endod.* **1998**, *86* (6), 707–714.
26. Jing, W.; Xuan, M.; Lin, Y.; Wu, L.; Liu, L.; Zheng, X. et al. Odontogenic Tumours: A Retrospective Study of 1642 Cases in a Chinese Population. *Int. J. Oral Maxillofac. Surg.* **2007**, *36* (1), 20–25.
27. Luo, H. Y.; Li, J. J. Odontogenic Tumors: A Study of 1309 Cases in a Chinese Population. *Oral Oncol.* **2009**, *45*, 706–711.
28. Mosqueda-Taylor, A.; Ledesma-Montes, C.; Caballero-Sandoval, S.; Portilla-Robertson, J.; Ruíz-Godoy Rivera, L. M.; Meneses-Garcia, A. Odontogenic Tumors in Mexico: A Collaborative Retrospective Study of 349 Cases. *Oral Surg. Oral Med. Oral Pathol. Oral Radiol. Endod.* **1997**, *84* (6), 672–675.
29. Willis, B. C.; duBois, R. M.; Borok, Z. Epithelial Origin of Myofibroblasts During Fibrosis in the Lung. *Proc. Am. Thorac. Soc.* **2006**, *3* (4), 377–382.
30. Daley, T. D.; Wysocki, G. P.; Pringle, G. A. Relative Incidence of Odontogenic Tumors and Oral and Jaw Cysts in a Canadian Population. *Oral Surg. Oral Med. Oral Pathol.* **1994**, *77* (3), 276–280.
31. Zegarelli, E. V.; Kutscher, A. H.; Napoli, N.; Iurono, F.; Hoffman, P. The Cementoma: A Study of 230 Patients with 435 Cementomas. *Oral Surg. Oral Med. Oral Pathol.* **1964**, *17* (2), 219–224.

CHAPTER 8

RELEVANT CURRENT APPLICATIONS OF INTERNET OF THINGS (IoT) IN BIOMEDICAL ENGINEERING

ANISH KUMAR

Computer Science and Information Technology, Institute of Technical Education and Research (ITER), Siksha 'O' Anusandhan Deemed to be University, Bhubaneswar, Odisha, India

ABSTRACT

Emerging IoT in this new era has brought lot of new technologies and devices in our day to day life. Now it's high time we should look forward and move towards its relevant current application in Biomedical industry. In this chapter we'll briefly discuss about the current situation and challenges present in Application of IoT in Biomedical Engineering.

8.1 INTRODUCTION

Here, IoT stands for "Internet of Things" concisely speaking that connecting of any device through the net in order that those devices will exchange information with one another on a network easing the lifetime of an individual. IoT is any device (mobiles, laptops, home devices, and anything used in daily life which is embedded with sensors).

With any quite in-built sensors with the flexibility to collect and transfer information through an online network while no manual intervention. The implanted innovation inside the article causes them to act with inside states and consequently the outside environment, which progressively helps in the determinations-making strategy. The IoT devices will produce data regarding individual's behaviors then analyze it, and will take action.[1]

More than nine billion "Appliances" square measure by and by associated with the web, starting at now inside the near future, this assortment is anticipated to ascend to a clobbering twenty billion.

In attention, IoT plays an important role in maintaining thousands of patient's information processed and helps them to capture their information anytime they require. To stay tabs on the placement of medical devices, patients, and personnel, several hospitals uses net of things.[1]

With the advancement in technology, today some hospitals implement good beds which will notice after the square measure occupied and once a patient is making an attempt to leave. It will simply adjust and ensures correct support and pressure to the patient while there will be no necessity for nurses. In attention, this good technology proves to be associate degree quality with home medication dispensers to mechanically transfer information to the cloud. As we all know IoT changing into slowly and slowly desegregation a part of our lifestyle includes attention. To create products or services a lot of economical and accessible, several attention suppliers or corporations use connected devices and applications.

Wearables like good watches, fitness trackers etc., and attention apps can permit patients and attention professionals to be in grips with alternatives. Doctors examine documents and resources instantly while not visit a library through medical reference material like Google glass, biometric stamp, lenses, etc. These devices facilitate attention suppliers to observe patient health remotely exploitation sensors, mobile communication devices, and actuators. These devices square measure referred to as the web of things for Medical devices or IoT-MD.[2]

8.1.1 BIRTH OF IoT

The term "The Internet of Things" (IoT) was given by Kevin Ashton in Proctor & Gamble in 1999. He's a co-founder of MIT's Auto-ID research lab. He pioneered RFID (used in Universal Product Code detector) for the supply-chain management domain. He conjointly started Zensi, an organization that produces energy sensing and observance technology.

Prior in 1982, the idea of the system of reasonable gadgets was referenced, with a changed Coke appliance at "Carnegie Andrew William Mellon University" that turned into the essential Internet-associated apparatus. This machine had the option to report its stock and whether or not recently loaded drinks were cold, once more in In 1994 Reza Raji explained the thought of IoT as tiny packets of information to an oversized set of nodes; therefore, on integrating and changing everything from home appliances to entire factories.[3]

8.1.2 BENEFITS OF IoT

The IoT may be a new net-like affiliation of technology publicized because of the next generation revolution—implying radical modification, disruption, and a completely new paradigm for the society. Specifically, the web of Things is associated with extension of the present connections digitally connected "things."

These things live and report information. This information is straightforward numbers from a stationary or mobile detector (such as a temperature sensor), or additional advanced findings from devices that live and report multiple information streams promptly.

These advanced devices will even actuate the information measurement (a connected thermostat is a simple example).

The IoT or web of Things may be a quickly growing topic in the market of late. Like each contemporary thought, the plenty are not too acquainted with this idea. It describes a scenario wherever human action with one another with none inter-human or human-to-machine interaction. Apart from the actual fact that it is a path-breaking discovery, it can even convince be very useful in facilitating our lives to manifolds.

Every new technology faces 1,000,000 challenges in its initial phases. Web of Things conjointly poses some grave problems that require to be tackled well so as to utilize its fullest potential. However, let's leave the threats aside for the present and focus solely on the positivity.

- **Improved Client Engagement**—IoT improves client expertise by automating the action. For example, any issues within the automobile are mechanically detected by the sensors. The driver similarly because of the manufacturer is notified regarding it. Until the time driver reaches the station, the manufacturer can check that the faulty half is obtainable at the station.
- **Improvisation of Technologies**—IoT has helped loads in increasing technologies and creating them higher. The manufacturer will collect information from completely different automobile sensors

and analyze them to enhance their style and build them far more economical.
- **Reduced Waste**—Our current insights area unit superficial, however, IoT provides time period info resulting ineffective deciding & allocation of resources, as instance, suppose a manufacturer suffer fault in multiple parts of device, he will check the running of these faulty parts of the device and may rectify the problem with producing belt.[2]

8.1.2.1 PRACTICAL APPLICATIONS

The versatility of IoT has become very fashionable in recent years. There are several benefits to having a tool supported IoT. There are numerous applications are out there within the market in several areas.

- **Medical and Healthcare:** Remote well-being perception and crisis warning framework are tests of IoT inside the restorative field.
- **Health Fix Health Monitor:** It will be utilized for the patient WHO can't go to specialists, material belonging them get chart, pulse, rate, skin temperature, body pose, fall identification, and action readings remotely. Electronic toll grouping framework is that the most accommodating model during this space.
- **Personal Home Automation System:** Home Automation framework is that the significant model during this space.
- **WeMo Switch reasonable Plug:** It is the chief accommodating gadget that associated with the home gadgets inside the Switch, a reasonable attachment. It connects to a regular outlet, acknowledges the office link from any gadget, and may want to flip it on and off on hit a catch on your cell phone.
- **Enterprise:** Within the venture space, a few applications are there like ecological perception framework, reasonable setting, and so forth.
- **Nest reasonable Thermostat:** it is associated with the web. The Nest adapts precisely your family's schedules and can precisely change the temperature bolster your exercises, to shape your home a great deal of affordable. There is conjointly a versatile application that allows the client to alter temperature and timetables.

- **Utilities:** Reasonable metering, brilliant network, and water perception framework are the preeminent supportive applications inside the various utility spaces.
- **Energy Management:** Advanced Metering Infrastructure is that the significant model during this space.
- **Massive Scale Deployment:** There are numerous massive comes in progress within the world. Songdo (South Korea), the primary of its kind totally wired sensible town, is close to completion. Everything during this town is planned to be wired, connected associate degree became an information stream that might be monitored by an array of computers without human interaction.[1]

8.1.3 FUTURE SCOPE FOR IoT

In the future, we can be able to even expect that individuals will opt for the property over security. As connecting with society, friends, and new technology with convenience can become a vital necessity. Individuals can even begin keeping all their data knowledge of themselves and their families in these devices, and that they begin commerce the security and security for the convenience. The users can begin creating all the rational calls at a very stake of their security and safety.

The kids, adults, and everybody can get addicted, and therefore, the house can become a giant IoT device. By 2025, it's calculable that there'll be over to twenty one billion appliances related to IoT.

A brisk recollect demonstrates any place gadgets are available and being used. As a fact in the year 2016, there have been more than 7 billion things connected to the web, in step with IoT Analytics. The market can increase to just about 11.6 billion IoT devices.[4]

8.1.3.1 CYBERCRIMINALS CAN IN ANY CASE USE IOT DEVICES TO ENCOURAGE DDOS ASSAULTS

In 2016, the globe was acquainted with the essential "Web of Things" malware—a strain of vindictive package that may contaminate associated with gadgets like DVRs, surveillance cameras, and the sky is the limit from there. The Mirai malware got to the gadgets abuse default parole and user names.

What occurred straightaway? The malware transformed the influenced gadgets into a botnet to encourage a Distributed Denial of Service (DDoS) assault that plans to overpower sites with web traffic. The assault all over up flooding one among the most significant site facilitating firms inside the world, transportation a spread of real, definitely gotten locales and organizations to an end for a significant long time.

This express strain of malware is named "open supply," which infers the code is offered for anybody to switch.

8.1.3.2 MANY DEVELOPING CITIES CAN PROGRESS TOWARD ACHIEVING "KEEN"

Buyers won't be the sole ones maltreatment IoT devices. Urban people group and organizations can sensibly grasp sensible progressions to keep away from lounging around inactively and cash.

That infers urban networks will be made to change, supervise from anywhere, and assemble information via components like visitant stands, camcorder police examination systems, bike rental stations, and taxis.

8.1.3.3 ARTIFICIAL LEARNING CAN IN ANY CASE TRANSFORM INTO A MUCH PROGRESSIVELY VITAL FACTOR

Sharp indoor house access, glowing infrastructure, and small producers amass learning on their affinities and occurrences of usage when we began voice-controlled contraptions, we grant them to get what we counsel them and save those records inside the cloud. Standard talking, the data are amassed to help motivate what's referred to as AI.

Computer-based intelligence may be a sort of programming designing that empowers PCs "to learn" while not someone programing them. The Personal Computers are tweaked in such a way that spotlights on discovering that they get. This upcoming information will by then empower the appliance to "acknowledge" the tendencies and maintains balance according to itself along these lines. For example, at the point when a video site proposes a flick you may like, it's presumably taken in your propensities kept up your past choices.[5]

Relevant Current Applications of Internet of Things   213

8.1.3.4   ROUTERS CAN IN ANY CASE BECOME MORE SECURE AND MORE INTELLIGENT

Since most client IoT devices live inside the home and can't have security pack put on them, they will be vulnerable to ambushes. Why? heaps of makers work to actuate their IoT item to progress quickly, thus security could similarly be associated in Nursing bit of knowing the past. This can be wherever the house switch accepted a very fundamental activity. The switch is, in a general sense, the entry explanation behind the web into your home. While a couple of your related devices can't be guaranteed, the switch can make protection at the entry reason. A standard switch gives some security, like parole protection, firewalls, and thus the ability to set up them to solely enable bound devices on your framework. Switch makers can probably still obtain new habits by which to support up security.

8.1.3.5   5G NETWORKS CAN REGARDLESS FUEL IOT ADVANCEMENT

Genuine remote bearers can even now strive off the 5G technology organizes in the year 2019. The technology of 5G—fifth-generation technology—ensures greater velocity and in this way the limit view extra sensible contraptions at unfaltering time.

Snappier structures mean the data collected by your reasonable contraption will be accumulated, broke down, and comprehends how to prevalent degree. That may fuel advancement at firms that manufacture IoT contraptions and lift client enthusiasm for crisp out of the container new item.

8.1.3.6   VEHICLES CAN GET SIGNIFICANTLY INCREASINGLY SPLENDID

The arrival of 5G can replace the vehicle work into a predominant rigging. The event of driverless cars—moreover in light of the fact that the related vehicles starting at now out in the town—can like getting the hang of moving quicker.

You likely won't consider your vehicle as an online of Things contraption. At any rate, new cars can coherently stall your knowledge and partner with choice IoT contraptions—similarly as elective front line vehicles on four wheels.

8.1.3.7 5G'S ARRIVAL WILL OPEN THE DOOR TO NEW INSURANCE AND SECURITY CONSIDERATIONS

In time, extra 5G IoT contraptions can be related to the 5G sort out than by methods for a Wi-Fi switch. This pattern can fabricate those gadgets extra powerless to direct assault, in venture with an ongoing Symantec journal post.

For home clients, it'll become more diligently to watch all IoT gadgets because of they'll sidestep a focal switch.

On a more extensive scale, the increased dependence on cloud-based capacity can offer assailants new focuses to intend to rupture.

8.1.3.8 IoT-BASED DDOS ASSAULTS CAN ASSAULT EXTRA RISKY STRUCTURE

Botnet-powered DDoS attacks have used infected IoT devices to bring down websites. IoT devices are often accustomed direct alternative attacks, in step with a Symantec diary post.

For instance, there could also be future makes an attempt to change IoT devices. A doable example would be a nation closing down home thermostats in Associate at Nursing enemy state throughout a harsh winter.

8.1.3.9 SECURITY AND PRIVACY CONSIDERATIONS CAN DRIVE LEGISLATION AND REGULATIVE ACTIVITY

The increase in IoT devices has simply one reason that is security and privacy considerations are rising.

In mid-2018, the EU Union enforced the final knowledge Protection Regulation. GDPR has crystal rectifier to similar security and privacy initiatives in many nations around the world. In the USA, Golden State recently passed a more durable privacy law.[6]

8.2 RELATED WORK

The exceptionally enormous issues that R&D group confronted were not exclusively to propose new checking devices, anyway also to give partner verification that can deal with all unique IoT gadgets. The designs for authentication, which work for cells, will be utilized to bear witness to various assortments of gadgets having sensors and microchips. The two fundamental sorts of contraptions of special security goals are proposed: hard source ensured goals-based validation sol. Physical verifying strategy is intended to shield devices from being broken or harmed on the progression of equipment layer by starting new thoughts. Elective side, steganography based for the most part is fundamentally the verification method that is planned and dependent on IoT radio recurrence ID devises (RFID) gadget character security field. It's pleasant security alternatives; a few calculations have as of late been arranged bolstered IoT RFID. IoT gadgets have limited assets and these gadgets square measure associated with the net. These open these gadgets to huge assortment of assaults and manufacture it powerless. Verification is expected to ensure security and decide characters to stop assaulter and pernicious assaults. Antiquated systems confirmation procedures and strategies need high assets concerning process. IoT is thought of a stressed asset setting any place procedure and vitality assets square measure limited. A light weight weight confirmation procedure with durable safety efforts is expected to save vitality and work process abilities. In this way during this postulation, we will propose a durable and lightweight weight verification method to fulfill the needs of IoT setting and supply a strong safety effort to stop noxious assaults and safeguard its protection.

Most recent anticipated verification systems have utilized totally various instruments to offer secure correspondence. Methods use HTTP conventions for confirmation correspondence experience the ill effects of high overhead came about because of exploitation HTTP convention that is not upgraded for asset confined IoT air. Various methods are used AES for correspondence steganography. AES uses long steganography keys and complex estimation that brought about high power utilization and won't work the necessities of IoT confined vitality assets.[7,8]

Various calculations have been anticipated to offer authentication for IoT gadgets. An Associate in Nursing expanded common authentication model has been anticipated for IoT air. They anticipated in a few improvements to the algorithmic program of validation of Challenge-reaction based for the most part RFID verification convention for circulated data atmosphere. They made it extra suitable to IoT the executives' framework air. Their procedure has three primary advances: include reinforcement gadget for each terminal gadgets utilized for predominant, add screen gadgets to pursue and screen terminal gadgets and finally include a push in caution component for fearsome for any fruitless authentication technique. In two-stage Attestation Protocol for Wireless gadget Networks in Distributed IoT Applications has been anticipated. This convention is an endorsement based generally confirmation method, two section validations empower each IoT gadgets and the administration station to guarantee and recognize each other, a protected association is built up and learning is moved solidly. They utilized convention underpins asset confinement of gadget hubs and takes into idea organize quantifiability and non-consistently. Endorsement specialist (CA) has been acclimated issue declarations. Existing hubs will move and change their area once they get their own declaration. CA will approve sensors character and speak with various substances of the system. System individuals to instate an association, they interface with the CA leading to check goal personality. This procedure is considered as Associate in Nursing completion to complete application layer validation method and relies upon various lower layer safety efforts. In Secure confirmation topic for IoT and cloud servers are anticipated, this blueprint essentially relies upon Elliptic Curve Steganography (ECC) based generally calculations that support higher security arrangements once it is contrasted and distinctive Public Key Steganography (PKC) calculations because of its minor key size. This verification convention utilizes Common Market for implanted gadgets that utilization HTTP convention. Exploitation the treats of HTTP to affirm reasonable gadgets might be a novel procedure. These gadgets might want to be structured with TCP/IP. The anticipated verification convention is proposed to utilize HTTP treats that are implemented to suit installed gadgets that have unnatural situations and constrained by cloud servers. The anticipated convention has three principle parts Registration stage, Pre-registered and login part and verification part. In enlistment part, the inserted gadgets are enrolled with the cloud server and it progressively transmits a treat that is hanged on the installed gadgets. In Pre-calculation and Login part, the gadgets before associating with the server might want to send a login demand. At long last, the authentication part each implanted gadget and cloud server correspondingly guarantee each extraordinary exploitation Common Market algorithmic program. Regardless of Common Market algorithmic program includes a minor steganography key anyway it will expand the size of the encoded message extensively. ECC algorithmic program is likewise extra progressed and harder to execute than various crypto graphical calculations and required extra procedure assets. In Threshold Steganography-based bunch Attestation (TCGA) subject for the IoT is anticipated. This model gives believability to all IoT gadgets dependent on group correspondence model. TCGA is expected to be implemented for Wi-Fi air. It makes a mystery channel or session key for each bunch verifications and it can likewise be utilized for group application. Each group has a bunch head that is liable for key age and conveying these new keys at whatever point once another group part is further to safeguard bunch key run this bunch head is alluded to as group specialist. Anticipated algorithmic program has five principle modules: key conveyance, key update, bunch credit age, verification examiner, and message mystery composing. SEA that might be a Secure and efficient Attestation and Authorization plan for IoT-based guide exploitation reasonable Gateways. This structure essentially relies upon testament-based DTLS affirmation convention. This plan incorporates the accompanying fundamental parts: therapeutic gadget organizes that assemble information from licenses body or rooms to aid treatment technique and medicinal ID. The subsequent part is reasonable E-Health course that licenses shifted framework correspondence and goes about as transitional for MSN and furthermore the web. The third half is Back-End System that gets procedures and stores gathered information. In a lightweight common authentication outline has been arranged, this pattern approves the characters of IoT gadgets took part in the situations before partaking in the system. They arranged decreased correspondence overhead influenced Application Protocol (CoAP) has been picked as underneath layer convention for giving correspondence between IoT gadgets. Validation is finished abuse the 128-piece Advanced encoding typical (AES). The character of the buyers and server is preeminent known. At that point, it gives totally various assets to the buyers' upheld explicit conditions decided in the solicitation. The restrictive explicit learning transmission decreased the transmitted parcels go which finishes in lessening vitality utilization and calculation. Data measure usage of the demonstration is also reduced and arranged another CoAP plausibility. The CoAP that works at the application layer gives the capacity to recover learning from gadgets like data and its gadget estimations. The fluctuated continuous applications are used these informations. Be that as it may, for the most part, it's a security request to not recover crude correspondence learning. Anyway exclusively deliberations, just as abnormal state condition of the found substances. Notwithstanding the idea of the asset influenced gadgets which may be gotten to by anybody on the net, vitality utilization decrease component assumes an essential job. Arranged instrument adds to these two needs which may prompt abnormal state states formation of readings the crude gadget. The arranged probability decreases the messages go once insightful a gadget asset which may bring about vitality utilization decrease and expanding timespan of the gadget.[9]

In a lightweight, common verification pattern has been arranged, this construction approve the personalities of IoT gadgets took part in the conditions before participating in the system. This arranged reduced CoAP has been picked as underneath layer convention for giving correspondence between IoT gadgets. Validation is finished abuse the 128-piece ordinary AES. The personality of the buyers and server is principal known. At that point, it gives totally various assets to the buyers' bolstered explicit conditions decided in the solicitation. The contingent explicit information transmission diminished the transmitted bundles run which finishes in lessening vitality utilization and calculation. The data measure use of the demonstration is also reduced and planned a new CoAP possibility. The CoAP that works at the application layer gives the capacity to recover learning from gadgets like data and its gadget estimations. Different constant applications are used these informations. But, generally it's a security demand to not retrieve raw communication knowledge. However, solely abstractions as well as high level state of the discovered entities. Notwithstanding the idea of the asset influenced gadgets which may be gotten by anybody on the net, vitality utilization decrease instrument assumes a fundamental job arranged instrument adds to these two needs which may prompt abnormal state states making of readings the crude gadget. Planned possibility reduces the messages range once perceptive a device resource which might result in energy consumption reduction and increasing time period of the device.[8,9]

8.2.1 LITERATURE SURVEY

With the passage of your time and development of society, individuals acknowledge that health is that the basic condition of promoting economic development. Some individuals say that existing public health service and its supportability are greatly challenged with reference to time. Worldwide the Government and trade are finance billions of bucks for the development of IoT computing, and a few of those comes embody China's National IoT set up by Ministry of trade and IT, European analysis Cluster on IoT (IERC), Japan's u-Strategy, UK's Future net Initiatives and Italian National Project of Netergit. The IoT applications within the field of medical and healthcare can profit patients to use the simplest medical help, shortest treatment time, low medical prices, and most satisfactory service. A scope of sensors that is snared to the body of a patient will be acclimated get wellbeing information immovably, and furthermore the gathered learning will be investigated (by applying some significant calculations) and sent to the server exploitation totally unique transmission media 3G/4G with base stations or Wi-Fi that is associated with the Internet. All the medicinal experts will access and consider the data, accept call subsequently to deliver benefits remotely. The technology will offer an oversized quantity of information concerning human, objects, time and area. Though joining this net innovation and IoT gives a larger than usual amount of zone and imaginative administration bolstered low-valued sensors and remote Communication. IPv6 and Cloud registering advance the occasion of combination of net and IoT. It's giving a great deal of possibilities of data accumulation, preparing, port administration, and diverse new administrations. Everything that partners with IoT needs a novel area or recognizing evidence which might be rehearsed with the assistance of IPv6. Utilization of the net of Things is film-capable and open outcomes to empowering the welfare applications to serve patients with higher treatment, correspondingly finished with the remote patient checking and stunning accommodating data managing. There are different moved attributes are depended upon to finish the medicative organizations advantage inside the earth displayed their own one of a kind arrangement for Remote Monitoring maintained IOT, blend of various structures like facility structure, organizations supplier system, Context Management Framework, content Systems and Environment Integration Platform. This plan utilizes RFID, wireless individual gadgets, implanted frameworks,

Monere and Movital equipment, 6LoWPAN, HDP, and the first important, a novel convention known as YOAPY. The arranged convention appears to be encouraging; at the same time, it doesn't legitimize the treatment of crisis things arranged a phonetics learning model to store and access the IoT information. The arranged framework, known as UDA-IOT, features anyway it's used in emergency restorative administrations. They actualize the DSS (choice emotionally supportive network) to disentangle the crisis issues created 6LowPAN-based omnipresent human services framework known as U-medicinal services that plays out the well-being recognition in each indoor and outside condition. The framework utilizes a live spilling stage for perusing of remote observing sensors of graphical record and temperature. The structured framework will store the apparent learning at remote server and utilize free Cloud administration like Ubuntu One. The proposed framework utilizes totally various gadgets and advances like switch, PC, IPv6, Serial Line net Protocol (SLIP), 3G/4G, Microcontroller MSP430 and CC2420, Tiny OS and Contiki Open supply bundle, ISR, and Wi-Fi. The proposed framework is fit to on-line gushing once the web speed is great, conjointly in crisis conditions. Blessing new structure for Remote recognition bolstered IoT and utilizes another convention known as YOAPY. The arranged framework is fit to constantly screen the patient well-being. There are people wherever the globe whose well-being may endure because of they don't have arranged access to successful well-being recognition. In any case, little amazing remote arrangements associated with the IoT are as of now making it potential for recognition to return to those patients as opposed to the other way around. These arrangements will be acclimated solidly catch quiet well-being information from a scope of sensors, apply complicated algorithms to research the information so share it through wireless property with medical professionals United Nations agency will build acceptable health recommendations.[8,9]

8.3 APPLICATION OF IOT IN BIOMEDICAL ENGINEERING

The IoT technology is turning into more and more common within the aid business. The first applications of IoT within the field of intelligent drugs includes the mental image of fabric management, digitization of medical info, and digitization of the medical processes.[10]

IoT basically incorporates of physical articles that square measure put in with sensors, actuators, process contraptions, and learning correspondence aptitudes. These square measures associated with frameworks for information transportation. Imagine a situation any place patient's therapeutic profile, imperative parameters, and dialyzer data square measure got with the assistance of empowering devices associated with his body. The patient doesn't need to be constrained to move from working environment to work environment to incite treatment. Or on the other hand perhaps, he will finish his subjective investigation the assistance of an adaptable home machine implied for the clarification data gathered from this apparatus is stony-poor down and place away, and in this way the aggregation from very surprising sensors and helpful contraptions chooses instructed determinations in advantageous procedure. Parental figures will screen the patient from any space and respond appropriately, in lightweight of the alert got. Moved treatment of this nature will fundamentally upgrade a patient's close to home fulfillment. The present degrees of progress in development and accordingly to the openness of the net form it possible to interface very surprising contraptions that may talk with each other and offer information. The Internet of Things (IoT) is another idea that grants customers to interface entirely unexpected sensors and clever contraptions to collect nonstop information from nature. The model named as "k-Social protection" makes usage of four layers; the gadget layer, the framework layer, the net layer and in this manner the organizations layer. All layers work together with each other suitably and capably to offer a phase to meaning to patients' prosperity information using propelled cell phones. The quick improvement of electronic devices, propelled cell phones, and tablets which might be conferred physically or remotely has turned into the vital gadget of step by step life. The exceptional back period of related world is web of Things (IoT) that interfaces devices, sensors, machines, vehicles, and diverse "things."[11]

8.3.1 AIMS AND SCOPE

Modern technologies of electronics promise an incredible impact within the field of aid. Miniaturization of electronic devices, at the side of progress in technology, knowledge science, and telecommunications, trigger new medicine applications resulting in a revolution in human drugs. Specific options of the future progress are:

- Personalization within the treatment with the individual wants and with the time evolving pathological configuration. Unprecedented preciseness within the diagnostic. Continuous health observation will offer semi-permanent info regarding the evolution of physiological indicators (e.g., vital sign, pulse, hypoglycemic agent level, EKG, etc.).
- At constant time, minimally invasive diagnosing is obtaining a lot of precise (e.g., oncology, etc.).
- In-vivo implantable devices become a reality: not solely they permit a permanent observation eventually related to the mandatory treatment (as an example, a lead-free pacemaker); however, within the close to future they will additionally accomplish to operate a missing or sick organ, like eye, kidney, or perhaps heart.

These progresses, typically selected by the term "telemedicine" or "e-health," square measure chiefly thanks to the evolution within the electronics and within the micro technologies. The miniaturization of size of the devices and a discount within the needed power for operation square measure the key enablers for implantable and wearable medicine devices. Additionally, progress within the "internet of things" technologies and within the processing permits a "big-data" aided technique to the diagnosing and health observation, also as a distant help to the persons having restricted autonomy.[12,13]

8.4 SPECIAL APPLICATIONS

The IoT innovation is changing into continuously normal inside the medicinal services exchange. The primary uses of IoT inside the field of shrewd medicine incorporates the picture of texture the executives, digitization of restorative information, and digitization of the therapeutic procedures. This innovation in medicinal services and a general apply of prescription gets expanded with the IoT framework. Experts reach is expanding inside an office. The shifted data gathered from huge arrangements of true cases will build each the exactness and size of medicinal data. The exactness of treatment conveyance is also improved by joining extra refined advances inside the human services framework. The IoT has opened a universe of prospects in medication: when associated with the net, standard medicinal gadgets will gather extremely valuable additional data, provide additional understanding into manifestations and patterns, change remote consideration, and usually give patients extra administration over their lives and treatment. The social insurance exchange is in a condition of pleasant sadness. Social insurance administrations zone unit costlier than any time in recent memory, total populace is maturing and furthermore the scope of perpetual maladies territory unit on an expansion. What we keep an eye on territory unit technique could be a world any place fundamental medicinal services would wind up distant to the dominant part, a curiously large segment of society would go inefficient because of adulthood and people would be extra obligated to endless infection, while innovation can't prevent the populace from maturing or destroy perpetual illnesses immediately, it will at least form human services simpler on a pocket and in term of availability. Restorative decisive exhausts a bigger than normal a bit of medicinal center bills. Advancement will move the calendars of remedial checks from a crisis center (restorative facility driven) to the patient's (home-driven). The most ideal task will reduce the need of hospitalization. The full scale use of this perspective in human administrations space could be a mutual desire as a result of it licenses helpful concentrations to play out extra suitably and patients to get higher treatment.

With the utilization of this development-based human administrations system, there are unit excellent focal points that may improve the standard and force of prescriptions and along these lines improve the quality of the patients. The IoT has been making authentic impact on each trade, and where this "advancement" sweptback by, you'll have the alternative to feel the limit. Right when the "disclosure" of web, IoT has been making waves that not one business inside the world will deny or confront. Those that do will be for quite a while deserted in light of the way that the test goes to end up more grounded and decided.

During this study, when all is said and done with exploring the engraving IoT that has made inside the social protection trade and the way in which it'll improve the lives of monstrous individuals around the globe. As per the reports introduced by the P&S displaying research, there'll be a compound yearly rate of improvement (CAGR) of thirty seven. About 6% inside the human administrations web of Things trade between the years 2015 and 2020. They ensure that this rising may be attributed to the perfect position of remote watching social protection systems which will find perpetual fundamental ailments.

By this, we will probably accept that IoT has steered and people can extravagant redid consideration for his or her well-being prerequisites; they will tune their gadgets to prompt them of their arrangements, calorie tally, practice check, weight level varieties and afterward rather more. Telemedicine observing primarily utilizes innovations related with the IoT innovation to make a patient-driven, remote meeting, and constant watching administration framework fixated on serving to fundamentally unwell patients. The underlying reason for arranging telemedicine watching innovation was proportional back the measure of patients getting into medical clinics and facilities.[10]

As indicated by the Centers for disorder the executives and bar (CDC), concerning 50% of US residents have at least one perpetual affliction, and their treatment costs represent more than 75% of the country's USD two trillion in therapeutic uses, moreover, to the high estimation of cutting edge treatment and medical procedure, specialists pay around billions of greenbacks on routine checks, research facility tests, and diverse watching administrations.

With the headway of telemedicine innovation, refined sensors are frequently acclimated screen patients with timeframe refreshes. In addition, the fundamental focal point of telemedicine watching has a tiny bit at a time moved from rising ways of life to rapidly giving conveyance information and to therapeutic projects fixated on scholastic trade.

In reasonable applications, well-being information of occupants is frequently transmitted through the net, rising the standard of restorative administrations. This innovation furthermore allows specialists to lead virtual meetings and supply scholarly help to various emergency clinics by masters from a larger than usual medical clinic. This can stretch out top notch therapeutic assets to essential human services foundations, encourage build up a semi-perpetual, nonstop training administration framework for clinical cases, and upgrade the standard of steady instruction for the essential social insurance staff.[11]

8.4.1 MEDICAL INSTRUMENTATION AND DRUG WATCHING AND MANAGEMENT

With the help of RFIDs, IoT has started to search out more extensive applications inside the field of restorative material administration picture. The IoT with RFIDs will encourage for maintaining a strategic distance from general medical problems by supporting inside the creation, conveyance, and pursue of medicinal gadgets and prescription. This will build the standard of therapeutic treatment though decreasing administration costs.

As indicated by the World Health Organization (WHO), the amount of fake meds inside the world adds up to very of offers of drug around the world. Learning from the Chinese Pharmaceutical Association demonstrates that, in China alone, at least 200 people kick the bucket every year as consequences of wrong or not reasonably utilized medicine. Between 11 and 26 years of patients utilize their meds mistakenly. This incorporates to a great extent of inaccurately recommended drugs.

Hence, RFID innovation can assume a significant job inside the pursuit and watching of drug and instrumentation and, in this manner, the guideline of the commercial center for medicinal item. In particular the IoT innovation inside the field of texture, the executives include applications inside the accompanying regions.[14,15]

8.4.2 THERAPEUTIC DEVICE AND PROFESSIONALLY PRESCRIBED MEDICATIONS ANTI-COUNTERFEITING

The name associated with an item can have a particular character that is remarkably irksome to fashion. This may assume a significant job in check of information and hostile to forging, demonstrating a productive countermeasure against restorative misrepresentation.

For instance, it'll be feasible to transmit sedate data to an open data from that a patient or medical clinic will check the substance of the name against the records inside the data to just decide potential fakes.

8.4.3 COMPLETE TIMEFRAME OBSERVING

From examination to flow, the total creation technique will use RFID labels to achieve thorough item viewing. This can be especially fundamental once the product gets dispatched. A pursuer put in on the sequential construction system will precisely decide each medication's data and transmit it to the data on the grounds that the item gets pre-bundled. All through the dispersion technique, any transitional information gets recorded whenever it implies that it's feasible to watch from completion to wrap up.

8.4.4 RESTORATIVE WASTE INFORMATION MANAGEMENT

Collaboration by clinics and transportation firms can encourage build up a discernible therapeutic waste pursue framework abuse RFID innovation. This may ensure that the medicinal waste gets appropriately shipped to the treatment organize and can stop the prohibited marketing of the biorisky restorative waste.

8.4.5 COMPUTERIZED HOSPITAL

Web of Things has expansive application prospects inside the field of therapeutic data board. At present the interest for restorative data, the board in medical clinics is particularly inside the accompanying angles: ID, test acknowledgment, and case history distinguishing proof. Recognizable proof incorporates quiet distinguishing proof, medico ID, test ID (counting drug ID), restorative instrumentation ID, lab ID, and case history ID (counting indications and ID of ailment).

We can isolate explicit applications into the ensuing regions:-

8.4.5.1 PATIENT INFORMATION MANAGEMENT

The patient's family therapeutic record, the patient's medicinal record, fluctuated examinations, restorative records, medicate hypersensitivities, and option electronic well-being documents will help specialists to create treatment programs. Specialists and attendants will live the patient's significant signs, and all through medicines like treatment, they will utilize timeframe watching information to wipe out the usage of wrong prescription or wrong needles which will precisely prompt attendants to hold out medication checks and elective work.

8.4.5.2 MEDICAL EMERGENCY MANAGEMENT

Their square measure some unprecedented conditions, at once their square measure mammoth quantities of losses, an Associate in Nursing failure to prevail in relations, or the fundamentally unwell. In such projections, RFID innovations' solid and practical stockpiling and testing ways can encourage with the quick distinguishing proof of significant subtleties like the patient's name, age, blood classification, crisis contact, and previous therapeutic record. This may accelerate confirmation techniques for crisis patients and leave extra valuable time for the treatment of unequivocal significance is that the establishment of 3G TV hardware in ambulances. As patients' square measure on their gratitude to the clinic, the medical clinic room is now acquiring acquainted with the patient's condition and may adequately indurate crisis salvage. In the event, the circumstance is amazingly stand-offish from the clinic, there's a shot of abuse remote therapeutic imaging frameworks as a piece of the crisis salvage technique.

8.4.5.3   DRUG STORAGE

RFID innovation will automatize the full chain of capacity, use, and examination to decrease the ideal working hours and shape forms that prior got directed on paper. It will encourage stop stock deficiencies and encourage the review of drugs. It likewise can encourage keep away from perplexity emerging from comparable medication names or portion amount and portion sort. In general, it'll fortify medication for the executives and ensure that drugs prepared instantly.

8.4.5.4   PATIENT INFORMATION MANAGEMENT

The use of RFID innovation to bank the executives will successfully stay away from the detriments of standardized tags having limited information capacity and may comprehend the objective of contact-less distinguishing proof, cut back blood pollution, comprehend multi-target recognizable proof, and improve learning arrangement intensity.

8.4.5.5   FIGHTING PHARMACEUTICAL ERROR

The data of the executives inside the drug store can encourage to ensure that medicine is appropriately conveyed and gotten. Until this point in time, drug store information the executives as of now gets upheld in such perspectives as giving solutions, altering measurements, nursing organization, understanding utilization of prescription, successfully following, stock administration, buy of gives conservation of ecological conditions, and assurance of period.

It is also to ensure which sort of medication gets endorsed to the patient, and to not exclusively record that medication the patient is taking and whether or not they've taken it anyway, even that the medication originated from. This maintains a strategic distance from the opportunity of patients missing planned meds, and inside the occasion of a top notch the board issue, influenced patients get known rapidly.

8.4.5.6 MEDICAL INSTRUMENTATION AND DRUG PURSUE

By precisely recording things and patient characters and giving tough help to mishap taking care of, out there restorative gadgets and prescription square measure represented. By precisely recording fundamental information like item use, antagonistic occasions, and territories any place inward control issues may happen, patients concerned and areas of unused item, we will track and deal with perilous item.

8.4.5.7 CONNECTED DATA SHARING

Initially, type a well-created and coordinated medicinal system through the sharing of restorative data and records. From one perspective, authorized specialists will check the patient's therapeutic record, history of ailment, treatment, and protection subtleties. Patients additionally will have the freedom to choose or supplant specialists and emergency clinics. On the contrary hand, town and provincial clinics will consistently associate with focal medical clinics for data and convenient expert suggestion, yet as course of action referrals and get training.

8.4.5.8 NEW BROUGHT INTO THE WORLD ANTI-KIDNAPPING SYSTEM

At an outsized general emergency clinic's OB and restorative strength office or a women and children's medical clinic, consolidating mother and child distinguishing proof administration, and infant security the executives can stop unattended access by pariahs. Exceptionally, each new-conceived should get an Associate in Nursing RFID anklet that unambiguously recognizes the child and envelops a particular correspondence with the mother's information. To check whether the family has the best possible infant, the RFID anklet exclusively should get checked by a medical attendant or elective staff member.

8.4.5.9 ALARM SYSTEM

Through timespan watching and pursue of emergency clinic therapeutic gadgets and patients, the framework can precisely request encourage inside the occasion of patient trouble. It'll furthermore prevent patients from deed the emergency clinic all alone and can encourage to stopping the damage or lawful offense of expensive gadgets and shield temperature-delicate prescription and research center examples.

8.4.6 RFID APPLICATIONS TO ASSIST THE OLDER LIVE SEVERALLY

Computer scientists at the University of State Capital, square measure is leading a project to develop the new RFID detector systems that support older individuals in order that they will safely keep freelance. Researchers used RFID and detector technology are used to spot and monitors people's activities mechanically. This will facilitate with each routine care Associate in Nursing emergency care within the case of an accident inside the house. In addition, the system options low input prices and no necessities for intensive testing within the face of an Associate in Nursing aging population, this application has a huge potential.[14,15]

8.4.7 SMART WHEEL-CHAIR APPLICATIONS

The task of good chair technology is to soundly and well deliver the user to a destination. During use, the chair not solely must settle for the user's instruction; however, it additionally must begin its obstacle turning away, navigation, and alternative practical modules in response to environmental info. Not like a self-driven mobile golem, the chair, and therefore, the user square measure is a cooperative system varied factors like style, safety, comfort, and simple operation square measure (or a minimum of ought to be) the foremost vital factors in good wheel-chair style.

Differences in potential users' physical capabilities mean that good-chair style should even be versatile and standard. Every user ought to be able to select the proper modules by their sort and degree of incapacity. Practical modules ought to be each removable and standardized, in order to that chair perform is modifiable as health levels modification.

The general perform of the good chair gets divided into the subsequent sub-functions: environmental perception and navigation functions, management functions, driving functions, and human–computer interaction. Through the practical analysis and modularization of the good wheel-chair's options plus specific analysis results, the system can probably incorporates three main parts: the detector Module, the Drive management Module, and therefore, the Human Interface Module.

The detector module would incorporates two components—internal state perception and external setting perception. The angle detector determines the angle and point info of the chair. The displacement speed and distance of the encoder provides the self-positioning info. Visual, ultrasonic, and proximity switches square measure chiefly chargeable for incessantly getting info concerning obstacles. For the drive management module, rear wheel configuration of a motor would get used with standard electric chair management operations—front, back, left, and right. Human–computer interaction is either finished physical controls, like a joystick or mouth stick or software package controls like a private laptop.

A smart chair has two freelance drive wheels, every equipped with a motor controller. The time period detection knowledge of the two motor controllers types the odometer relative positioning detector. The installation of the inclination detector; and therefore, the gyro is finished to live the posture state of the chair throughout the traveling method.

Ultrasonic sensors and proximity switches acquire close info. To realize a wider vary of obstacle info, eight infrared sensors, and eight supersonic sensors get equipped with the system. Also, installation of a CCD camera is finished to see the depth info before of the chair.

Additionally, the good chair will balance alone on two wheels. This delicacy needs that the chair gets designed with a singular structure supported the thought of driving every wheel by a separate DC motor and keeping the balance of the chair's weight directly higher than the wheels on one axis.

This gets achieved by utilizing sensors to see the pitch and yaw, thus, crucial the angle of the chair in time period. Signals from the sensors move to the chair's processor that runs the data through an effect rule to see the best speed and direction for every wheel to keep up balance whereas moving forward or backward.

The good chair uses a mix of a tilt detector Associate in Nursing a gyro to make an angle detector capable of crucial the wheel-chair's angle because it travels across a plane. The utilization of the lean detector is to see the wheel-chair's degree of deviation from vertical; whereas, the gyro determines its angular speed.

8.4.8 MOBILE MEDICATION

By mensuration significant signs, as indispensable sign and heartbeat rate, and shaping a private restorative profile for each patient just as bodyweight, steroid liquor level, muscle to fat ratio, and super atom content, we will examine the patient's general life and return physiological marker learning to the patient's locale, overseer, or associated medicinal association. This allows the patient to shape auspicious modifications to their eating regimen, encourages the age of opportune tweaked restorative suggestion, and gives investigation information to emergency clinics and examination foundations.

8.4.9 APPLICATIONS OF RFID WRISTBANDS

It won't be long before every person's telephone are going to be sort of a non-public doctor whereas everybody actually has their own expertise with these matters, it's not uncommon in China to visualize long lines of patients—waiting to require a number and see a doctor. Patients overcome by visits, as hospitals square measure flooded with thousands or tens of thousands of outpatients during a single day.

So, will this technique work? Once someone becomes unwell, he or she needs to visualize an Associate in Nursing professional. Hence, however, will we tend to expeditiously service everyone? This will be done exactly by encouraging these sorts of changes as we tend to enter the longer term expertise makes an Associate in Nursing professional, and this expertise is accumulated by observant knowledge indicators associated with the patient's malady.

If an Associate in Nursing expert's expertise is compiled into an information, then all the patient must do to enter his or her knowledge indicators into the system once the parameters within the information have reached a comfortable level, the information are going to be able to perform Associate in Nursing automatic diagnosing. In the end, the information becomes a form of "robot professional."

These databases work by aggregation Associate in Nursing adequate quantity of the expert's cancer cases, combining them to make knowledge indicators and, thus, generating an information model. As an example, if we've got the information indicators for the treatment of ten thousand cases of leukemia, then the information contains ten thousand solutions for treating leukemia.

This kind of information can eventually remodel into an inbuilt software package in our cell phones, increasing the quality of treatments. If the software package is unable to assess things expeditiously, then an individual's professional is going to be able to administer treatment over the net. In time, every folks can have his or her own "private golem doctor" residing on our phones.

8.4.10 *GPS POSITIONING APPLICATIONS FOR PATIENTS WITH CARDIOVASCULAR DISEASE*

Each person must build their health information. If a sufferer of cardiovascular disease has created their digital health file, then, as presently as their heart begins to behave abnormally or poses an on the spot risk, the relevant knowledge are going to be right away passed to the system which will use GPS positioning to decision the required emergency services from the closest hospital.

This may be a straightforward IoT application, but, within the future, we tend to might all have our own check-up devices reception. All we'd like to try and do is place our palm on the device which will then collect pressure, heart rate, pulse, and vital sign within the future; it would even be able to perform chemical tests.

This knowledge are going to be mechanically passed to the hospital's knowledge center, and, if necessary, a doctor can raise United States to come back into the hospital for additional analysis or move to a close-by treatment center to receive treatment.

8.4.11 HEALTH ID CARD

When we get onto the railway system, near to everything will get accomplished with the swipe of a card. This makes the complete expertise far more convenient for the bulk of users.

In medical IoT field, seeing a doctor ought to be like older the railway system. Over the course of medical treatment, the user's official ID card is that the solely legal proof of identity and should get scanned on a card reader, with the patient submitting a particular quantity of cash as a payment during a few seconds, the machine-driven card reader/writer will then turn out an Associate in Nursing "RFID Visit Card" (this may additionally double as an Associate in Nursing insurance card) that the patient will use to induce a number for seeing the doctor.

Once the patient encompasses a card, they will move to see a doctor at any treatment center. At the treatment center, the system can mechanically enter their info into the corresponding doctor's digital computer. Throughout treatment, info associated with the doctor supply examinations, medicine, and alternative treatment info gets passed on to the acceptable departments.

As long because the patient has their "RFID Visit Card," the cardboard reader/writer at the corresponding department will check all of this info, issue medication, and administer treatment while not requiring the patient to run back and forth calculative and creating payments. Once the procedure is complete, the fee printer prints out a receipt and price list.

Also associated with "RFID Visit Cards, hospitals shall be able to concede patients Associate in Nursing "RFID wristband" which is able to embrace the patient's name, gender, age, profession, arrival time, diagnosing time, examination time, and fee info. The accomplishment of getting the patient's identity info gets refrained from any manual entry; and therefore, the secret writing of patient's profiles is required to shield their privacy.

This ensures that the wristband is that the solely supply of the patient's identification info and avoids human error derived from manual entry. What is more, these wristbands also will embrace positioning practicality, creating it not possible for the user to leave of the hospital.

If a patient forcibly removes their "RFID wristband" or leaves a particular vary round the hospital, then the system can issue Associate in Nursing alert, triggering Associate in Nursing analysis of the wearer's very important signs (breathing, heart rate, pulse) and confirm the patient's "threat level" supported that info. The system are going to be able to assess physiological changes 24 h daily, and once the wearer's threat level reaches a particular threshold, Associate in Nursing alerts are going to be issued mechanically to permit hospital workers to reply as presently as doable.

Examination, imaging, surgery, drug administration, and alternative tasks common to the treatment method is all expedited by confirming patient info through their "RFID wristband" and recording the time that every step within the method begins. This ensures that nurses and hospital examination workers at each level administer the acceptable care while not error, thus, providing the standard of the complete treatment method.

The patient will use their "RFID wristband" to see their treatment fees and specific card reading machines. They will additionally print their fee results, insurance plans, rules and laws, nursing directions, treatment plan, and drug info. This may serve to extend the patient's ability to simply acquire their treatment info and increase overall patients' satisfaction.[15]

It can be further used in several fields such as[14]:

8.4.11.1 REAL TIME LOCATION TECHNOLOGY

Through IoT, doctors will use real-time location services and track the devices used for treating patients. Medical employees could typically keep the devices in out-of-sight areas that make them troublesome to search out once other medical employees come on the scene.

Therapeutic gear and gadgets like wheelchairs, scales, defibrillators, neutralizers, siphons, or perception instrumentation will be named with sensors and placed simply with IoT aside from real-time location services, there square measure IoT devices that facilitate in environmental observation similarly (checking the icebox temperature, for example).

8.4.11.2 ANTICIPATING THE ARRIVAL OF PATIENTS IN PACU

With the intervention of web of Things, clinicians will predict the arrival of patients UN agency square measure recuperating within the

Post-Anesthesia Care Unit (PACU). They'll additionally monitor the standing of patients in real time.

8.4.11.3 HYGIENE COMPLIANCE

There square measure hand cleanliness perception frameworks that may discover the level of tidiness in an exceedingly tending worker. Predictable with the center for disease the board and impedance inside us, in regards to one patient out of every twenty gets contaminations from absence of right hand cleanliness in medical clinics. Different patients lose their lives as after effects of medical clinic non-inheritable contaminations.

The collaborations inside the hand cleanliness perception frameworks square measure cleared out constant and if a specialist approaches a patient's bed while not clothing his hands, the gadget would start loud and that isn't every one of the information with respect to the tending worker, his ID, time, and site would all be able to be encouraged into a data and this data would be sent to the included experts.

8.4.11.4 EXACT COSTS AND IMPROVISING PATIENT EXPERIENCE

The tending business must watch out for the spending limit and at an equal time have refreshed foundation to create higher patient encounters. In view of the consistent connection between gadgets that IoT has made possible, it's at present feasible for the medicinal representatives to get to persistent data from the cloud insofar as they're hanging in there.

8.4.11.5 END-TO-END NETWORK AND MODERATENESS

The IoT will automatize patient consideration work stream with the help tending quality goals and option new innovations, and cutting edge tending offices.

The IoT in tending permits capacity, machine-to-machine correspondence, information trade, and learning development that makes tending administration conveyance compelling.

Network conventions: Bluetooth LE, Wi-Fi, Z-wave, ZigBee, and option elegant conventions, tending work force will change the method they spot medical issue and diseases in patients and may, moreover, present progressive manners by which of treatment.

Consequently, technology-driven setup brings down the price, by scaling down unnecessary visits, utilizing high equality resources, and rising the allocation and coming up with.

8.4.11.6 DATA ANALYSIS

The vast quantity of knowledge that a tending device sends terribly in very short time, thanks to their time period application is difficult to store and manage if the access to the cloud is unobtainable. Even for tending suppliers to amass knowledge devices and sources and analyze it manually may be a robust bet.

IoT gadgets will gather report and investigate the data in timespan and slice the necessity to store the information. This all will happen overcloud with the providers exclusively acquiring access to definite reports with charts.

Moreover, tending operations enable organizations to urge the important tending analytics and data-driven insights that speed up decision-making and are a smaller amount liable to errors.

8.4.11.7 TRACKING AND ALARMS

The on-time alarm is basic on the occasion of intolerable conditions. Restorative IoT gadgets assemble significant learning and move that information to specialists for timespan pursue, while dropping notices to people with respect to key fragments by methods for adaptable applications and alternative coupled devices.

Reports and alerts give a firm inclination two or three patient's condition, paying little heed to spot and time. It, moreover, empowers work to proficient choices and supply on-time treatment. Along these lines, IoT grants time allotment disturbing, after, and recognition, which licenses dynamic prescriptions, higher accuracy, and proficient mediation by authorities and improves all outpatient social protection movement results.

8.4.11.8　REMOTE THERAPEUTIC ASSISTANCE

In occasion of partner crisis, patients will contact a specialist UN organization is a few kilometers away with a shrewd versatile applications.

With quality arrangements in tending, the surgeons will in a split second check the patients and set up the diseases in a hurry.

Likewise, different arrangement chains that square measure forecast to make machines which will disperse medicine on the reason of patient's solution and affliction-related information available by means of coupled gadgets. IoT can improve the patient's consideration in medical clinic. Progressively, this can cut on individuals' scope on tending.

8.4.11.9　RESEARCH

The IoT for tending also can be used for analysis functions. It's as a result of IoT allows USA to gather a colossal quantity of knowledge regarding the patient's health problem which might have taken a few years if we tend to collected it manually. This knowledge, therefore, collected will be used for applied mathematics study that might support the medical analysis. Thus, IoT doesn't solely save time, however, additionally our cash which might go into the analysis.

Thus, IoT incorporates a nice impact within the field of medical analysis. It allows the introduction of larger and higher medical treatments.

IoT is employed in an exceedingly type of devices that enhance the standard of the tending services received by the patients.

Even the present devices square measure currently being updated by IoT by merely exploitation embedding chips of a wise device. This chip enhances the help and care that a patient needs originating from multiple problems.[9]

The objective is to deliver quality restorative guide to patients, and by payment a little low amount there on foundation, emergency clinics will give superb consideration to patients at modest rates. IoT plans to deliver higher patient adventure by:-

- Lighting of electrical through close to home administration
- Communicate to family and organization via email administrations
- Immediate thoughtfulness regarding patient needs.

8.4.12 REMOTE OBSERVING

Remote well-being perception is a pivotal use of web Of Things. Through perception, you'll have the option to offer satisfactory tending to individuals that square measure in desperate might want to encourage. With IoT, gadgets fitted with sensors apprise the included tending providers once there's any alteration inside the significant elements of somebody.

These contraptions would be prepared for applying pushed computations and analyzing them thusly the patient gets right thought and helpful guide. The accumulated patient information would be hold tight in cloud. Through remote discernment, patients will altogether diminish the length of restorative center keep and perhaps, even crisis facility re-attestation. This sort of intervention may be an assistance to individuals living alone, particularly seniors. If there's any impedance inside the consistently development of someone, alerts would be sent to relations and anxious prosperity suppliers. These recognition devices square measure accessible inside the kind of "wearables" too.

8.4.13 WORKING ON RESEARCH SIDE

Protein examination and creation investigation points of interest from web of Things. Through IoT, analysts' square measure prepared to break down the exactness of the instrumentation, and it rewards them by shortening their work course through quantitative and duplicable examination of proteins.

At the point when partner interminable exhibit of gadgets is associated, the tending business is prepared to create ascendible answers for its patients. Assortment of tending applications giving cutting-edge altered arrangements square measure released to them, which are as:

- Medication Dispensing Device by Philips—along these lines patients won't miss a portion any longer; useful for senior patients.
- Niox Mino by Aerocrine—for routine estimations of Intric synthetic compound in an exceedingly patient's breath.
- UroSense by Future Path Medical—for siphoned patients to see their center blood warmth and body waste yield.
- GPS Smart Sole—this is regularly a shoe-following wearable gadget for insanity patients UN office have the propensity for overlooking things.

8.4.14 SPECIALIZED ISSUES FACING MEDICAL IOT

In the therapeutic field, we will in general address a few specialized issues confronting IoT. These issues incorporate the following.[5]

8.4.14.1 DYNAMIC NETWORKING AND NODE QUALITY MANAGEMENT IN LARGE-SCALE NETWORKS

At the point when there's an Associate in Nursing development of the watching framework to cover up private networks, urban communities, or perhaps whole nations, the components of the system will be overpowering, and watching hubs and base stations alike can all get the chance to be versatile somewhat. In this way, we must style partner in Nursing relevant design the executives structure and system quality administration ways.

8.4.14.2 KNOWLEDGE COMPLETENESS AND DATA COMPRESSION

Hubs can for the most part get the opportunity to direct looking for 24 h every day, conglomeration a gigantic amount of information that must be hung on utilizing a pressure standard to curtail capacity and transmission volume. Be that as it may, antiquated learning pressure calculations square measure unreasonably expensive for locator hubs. Pressure calculations can't lose the main learning. Something else, the framework may misdiagnose the patient's condition.

8.4.14.3 DATA SECURITY

Remote identifier arrange hubs type a self-sorted out system that is powerless to assaults and is, clearly, dangerous once overseeing patient information that must be whole secret.

The processing intensity of a finder hub is remarkably short. Thus, antiquated security and mystery composing innovation aren't material to those outcomes. Along these lines, we will in general should style an Associate in Nursing mystery composing principle fitting to the abilities of a finder hub.

8.4.15 JOINING: NUMEROUS DEVICES

Joining of various contraptions conjointly causes obstacle inside the use of IoT inside the thought fragment.

The clarification behind this square is device makers that haven't accomplished an understanding concerning correspondence shows and common.

Along these lines but the inconstancy of gadgets zone unit associated; the refinement in their correspondence convention muddles and prevents the technique for learning total.

This non-consistency of the associated gadget's conventions hinders the all-out strategy and diminishes the extent of measure capacity of IoT in consideration.

8.4.16 INFORMATION OVER-BURDEN AND PRECISION

As referenced before, information collection is inconvenient in light of the work of different correspondence conventions and benchmarks.

In any case, IoT devices still record a lot of learning. The information accumulated by IoT contraptions domain unit used to achieve critical encounters. Regardless, the measure of learning is thusly colossal that explanation bits of information from it have ended up being hazardous for pros that finally impact the standard of essential initiative. Additionally, this stress is climbing as additional contraptions zone unit related that record extra and additional learning.

8.4.17 COST

Amazed to learn value worries inside the test areas? I do know the vast majority of you would be; anyway, the most reduced line is: IoT has not made the consideration encourages sensible to the individual in any case.

The blast inside the consideration costs might be a stressing sign for everybody especially the created nations.

The circumstance is such it offered ascend to "Restorative Tourism" during which patients with indispensable conditions access care offices of the creating countries which cost them as less as basic part. IoT in consideration as a thought idea plan a motivation might be an interesting and promising thought.

In any case, it has not settled the worth worries starting as of now. To with progress actualize IoT application improvement and to accomplish its complete enhancement the partners should construct it cost successful else it'll perpetually avoid everybody's scope aside from the people from the high class.

8.4.18 UTILIZATIONS OF IOT IN BIOMEDICAL

The rising of IoT is stimulating for everyone because of its absolutely interesting degree of usage in different territories. In thought it has various applications. IoT in thought helps in:-

- Reducing ER hold up time
- Tracking patients, staff, and stock
- Enhancing drug the board
- Ensuring openness of crucial equipment

IoT has conjointly presented numerous wearables and gadgets that have made existences of patients comfortable. These gadgets zone unit as pursues:

8.4.19 HEARABLES

Hearables zone unit new-age convenient speakers that have totally overhauled the strategies people that persevered through hearing issue move with the planet. Nowadays, hearables zone unit immaculate with Bluetooth that matches up your wireless with it.

It awards you to channel, equalization, and add superimposed choices to genuine sounds. Doppler Labs is that the most fitting instance of it.

8.4.20 INGESTIBLE SENSORS

Ingestible sensors are a unit really a bleeding edge science wonder. These are the unit pill-sized sensors that screen the solution in our body and alert us if it perceives any peculiarities in our bodies.

These sensors may be assistance for a diabetic patient since it would energize in edge reactions and supply with an early advised for diseases. Proteus Digital Health is one such model.

8.4.21 MOODABLES

Moodables locale unit perspective improving devices that energize in rising our attitude for the term of the day. It should sound like phantasy, at any rate it's immediately from this present reality.

Thync and Halo Neurosciences zone unit effectively connected on it and has made colossal advancement.

Moodables zone unit head-mounted wearables that send low-power current to the mind lift our perspective.

8.4.22 PC VISION INNOVATION

PC vision development along the edge of AI has offered rise to meander advancement that hopes to duplicate seeing and in this manner picking supported it.

Robots like Skydio use PC vision development to see tangles and to investigate around them.

This advancement may be used for ostensibly debilitated individuals to investigate with capability.

8.4.23 HEALTHCARE CHARTING

IoT devices like Audemix scale back abundant manual work that a doctor has got to do throughout patient charting.

It is high-powered by voice commands and captures the patient's knowledge.

It makes the patient's knowledge promptly accessible for review. It saves around doctors' work by 15 h per week.

8.5 CONCLUSION

Late advances in small scale electro-mechanical frameworks (MEMS) innovation, remote correspondences, and computerized material science have empowered the occasion of moderate, low-control, multi useful remote indicator hubs that are little in size and impart unbound quickly removes.[3,7,9] These little remote locator hubs that accommodates sensing, handling, and act parts, influence the idea of identifier systems bolstered the helpful exertion of a larger than usual assortment of hubs. The strength of emergency clinic representatives is collected by misuse some of these new available applications and apparatuses. Inside the guide field, issues like long-run patient consideration in medical clinics, support for senior people gathering and in a portable setting are being referenced inside the domain of remote finder systems. This proposal has given an inaccessible patient perception framework structure abuse remote identifier hubs fit for perception numerous totally various conditions: emergency clinics, home, and versatile. The structure maintained may be a period calm observation system that empowers restorative experts to look at their patients on a blocked off site, to watch their noteworthy signs and to give them some proposition to therapeutic guide meds. The structure made has the ensuing workplaces intercalary to positively affect productive and esteem feasibility by keeping the patients from re-hospitalization and discernment different patients' prosperity staying meanwhile.[7,9]

- The information is offered for reviewing on the central server, and may be gotten to remotely by infer that of a normal applications program. This checked net server abuses the instinctive conceivable outcomes of the net to mix the mixing of different sorts of clinical data with assistance of patient-provider correspondence, raising the likelihood of achieving progressively raised measures of patient thought.
- The in-network data collection system upheld in our plan partner degree endeavor to assemble the principal significant data from the sensors and transmits it to the base station in a vitality affordable way with least data dormancy. "In-organize" implies that causing mostly total qualities rather than crude qualities, in this way lessening force utilization.
- The harvest time discovery equation upheld, watches an adjustment in edges related to an intersection of a gathering quickening limit among steady measure. The enormous increasing speed along the edge of the adjustment of edge as to the underlying position among steady time period is marked as a fall. The 198 outcomes demonstrated that the recipe can possibly separate between a fall and every day schedule exercises.
- The sequential measurable examination topic utilizes a direct testing method to coordinate two sub groupings that are of different lengths.

Our outcomes demonstrate that the recipe created has higher precision in finding irregularities inside the ECG sign of the patients.
- The framework grew precisely cautions the doctors, crisis division work force-related parental figures once a peculiarity is identified through email and SMS administrations.

The gadget lattice configuration is expected and tried for observing totally various groups of patients: Remote watching of post-usable patients in emergency clinics, senior patients' gathering-related patients brimming with COPD and metallic component in ambulant surroundings to change period gadget data collection and thus the sharing of machine and capacity assets for gadget handling and the executives. The restorative server in our framework created has the consequent offices to deliver consistent access to a decent sort of assets in an extremely inescapable way.

1. To store the data gathered by the gadget hubs.
2. To encourage investigation with the help of associated agent's calculation controls and predicts the unwellness with the offered databases.
3. To alarm the doctors, crisis divisions, and overseers through email and SMS benefits once oddity occurs.
4. With its potential use inside the emergency clinics and private consideration fields, remote gadget systems have a significant job in the lives of 199 patients. Other than transferral solace to patients, there are gigantic mechanical edges inside the space of decreasing costs, rehospitalization, and up instrumentality and patient administration.

8.6 SCOPE FOR FUTURE APPLICATIONS

Wireless device networks, a widely known technology contain little, powered "motes" with restricted computation and radio communication capabilities. This technology has the potential to impact the delivery and study of resuscitative care by permitting important signs to be mechanically collected and totally integrated into the patients care record and used for period sorting, correlation with hospital records, and semi-permanent observation. This system innovation gives a vastly improved goal to remote watching of post-usable patients in a very clinic, senior patients gathering, and patients loaded with COPD and metallic component all through their restoration sum in ambulant conditions. There are a few distinct expansions potential to this work might be examined extra. The immediate augmentation is to utilize the software engineering in remote gadget systems to investigate the simple parallel dispersed calculation, appropriated capacity, data solidness, and car characterization of gadget readings to help the doctors inside the early elucidation of maladies. With gadget arranges nearly planning, security issues bearing on the gadget systems are inside the spotlight. Due to the affectability of medicinal data, sombre protection and security are inescapable for all segments of consideration frameworks. The second augmentation of this work is to consolidate security conventions to deliver security in gadget systems, with a weight on authentication, key administration and appropriation, secure steering, and ways for interruption recognition. Two hundred a few "standard" and restrictive conventions utilize the media-get to controller (MAC) and in this way the physical circuits (PHY) identified with IEEE 802.15.4 radios. Those conventions utilize their own courses of action of bits and bytes to move information between hubs; anyways none of them utilize the net Protocol (IP). So, they can't straightforwardly speak with Internet-based gadgets and net servers/programs. The IPv6 over Low power Wireless Personal space Networks (6LoWPAN) typical offers another because of it utilizes the IPv6 convention and may work similarly keep running over remote and wired associations. The third expansion is to fuse 6LoWPAN correspondences that needn't bother with an entire modify of partner IEEE 802.15.4 radio stack. Rather, 6LoWPAN includes partner adjustment layer that lets the radio stack and IPv6 interchanges work along. Remote gadget Actor Networks (WSANs) are ascending as a substitution age of gadget systems. In Wireless gadget Actor Networks, sensors assemble information concerning the physical world; while entertainers take choices thus perform pertinent activities upon the environment that licenses remote, machine-controlled interaction with the environment. The nearness of one instrument in gadget systems kills the need for the coordination and correspondence among actuators and a scantily associated system dispenses with the need for area the executives. The fourth augmentation is to fuse WSANs in remote viewing of patients to precisely incite the gadgets like the electronic gadget, medicate conveyance framework, muscle trigger, and so forth, when dangerous occasions happen. Our momentum work likewise can stretch out extra to watch sports characters and patients brimming with various explicit illnesses all through their conventional routine exercises.[7,9,16–18]

KEYWORDS

- IoT history
- IoT current scenario
- scope
- challenges
- devices and technology
- biomedical industry
- IoT application

REFERENCES

1. Mujadiya, N. *Chapter 1: Introduction to Internet of Things*, n.d. Retrieved 22 May 2019, from IoT with Raspberry Pi: https://medium.com/iot-with-raspberry-pi/chapter-1 z-introduction-to-internet-of-things-c8c459f4f961
2. Sinha, S. *Introduction to Internet of Things: IoT Tutorial with IoT Application*, May 22, 2019. Retrieved 12 June 2019, from Edureka: https://www.edureka.co/blog/iot-tutorial/
3. Aayush. *Internet of Things (IoT): Introduction, Applications and Future Scope*, June 19, 2017. Retrieved 10 June 2019, from GMKIT: http://www.gkmit.co/articles/internet-of-things-iot-introduction-applications-and-future-scope#
4. Curtin University (CurtinX). *Introduction to the Internet of Things (IoT)*, n.d.. Retrieved 24 May 2019, from edX: https://www.edx.org/course/introduction-to-the-internet-of-things-iot-1
5. Thought Leadership. *IoT in Healthcare: Scope, Future and Challenges*, 23 Feb 2018. Retrieved 11 June 2019, from T&VS: https://www.testandverification.com/thought-leadership/iot-in-healthcare-scope-future-and-challenges-23-feb-2018/
6. Peerbits. *Internet of Things in Healthcare: Applications, Benefits, and Challenges*, n.d. Retrieved 15 June 2019, from Health & Fitness Iot: https://www.peerbits.com/blog/internet-of-things-healthcare-applications-benefits-and-challenges.html
7. Shodganga. *Conclusion and Future Work*, n.d.. Retrieved 12 June 2019, from https://shodhganga.inflibnet.ac.in/bitstream/10603/35507/12/12_chapter%207.pd
8. Mustafa Abdullah Azzawi, K. A. A Review on Internet of Things (IoT) in Healthcare. *Int. J. Appl. Eng. Res.*, 2016.
9. Peeyush, A. B. *Internet of Things: A Review on its Future Scope & Challenges*; National Conference on Recent Advancement in Engineering & Science, 2015.
10. Diksha, B.; Wasankar, D. V. Application of Internet of Things in the Field. *Int. J. Innov. Res. Comput.* **2017**.

11. Ian Rubín de la Borbolla, M. C. *Applying the Internet of Things (IoT) to Biomedical Development for Surgical Research and Healthcare Professional Training*, 2017. Retrieved from IEEE: https://ieeexplore.ieee.org/abstract/document/7998399
12. Elsevier, 2017. https://www.journals.elsevier.com/microelectronics-journal/call-for-papers/special-issue-on-internet-of-things-for-biomedical-applicati
13. Christopher, G. *Internet of Things in Healthcare: What's Next for IoT Technology in the Health Sector*, July 19, 2016. Retrieved 10 June 2019, from ComputerWorldUK: https://www.computerworlduk.com/iot/iot-centred-healthcare-system-3643726/
14. Tatiana Huertas, D. M. Biomedical IoT Device for Self-Monitoring Applications. *IFMBE Proceedings*, 2017.
15. Thahir, S. *6 Applications of IoT in the Healthcare Industry*, Feb 10, 2016. Retrieved 17 June 2019, from CABOT: https://www.cabotsolutions.com/2016/02/applications-iot-healthcare-industry
16. Aeris Blog. *The Future of IoT Medical Monitoring*, Jan 19, 2017. Retrieved 13 June 2019, from Aeris Blog: https://blog.aeris.com/the-future-of-iot-healthcare-monitoring
17. Patient, M. D. *IoT in Healthcare: Scope, Future and Challenges*, 2018. Retrieved 13 June 2019, from Steemit: https://steemit.com/health/@patientmd/iot-in-healthcare-scope-future-and-challenges
18. Srivastava, S. *Possibilities of IoT Application in the Healthcare Sector*, Feb 1, 2019. Retrieved 20 June 2019, from Appinventiv: https://appinventiv.com/blog/iot-in-healthcare/

INDEX

A

Advanced medical management
  Internet of Things (IoT), 46
    advanced smart medical, 49
    battling pharmaceutical error, 48
    medication storage management, 47–48
    persistent statistics management, 47
    quiet information management, 48
    restorative device and
      pharmaceuticals anticounterfeiting, 48–49
    smart medicinal management, 47
    therapeutic waste information management, 49
Analysis of efficiencies between EEG and MRI
  Internet of Things (IoT)
    brain–computer interface (BCI), 71
    critical survey, discussion, 72
    dataset used EEG recordings, 73–79
    depression, 70
    depression and machine learning, 81–83
    fMRI and EEG signals, 71
    machine learning (ML), model, 84–88
    machine learning (ML) techniques, 71
    seizure formation and depression, 80–81

B

Biomedical signal analysis, IoT
  body area network (BAN), 5
  cardiovascular disease (CVD), 3
  communication, 11
    Arduino setup, 12
    blood pressure, 18
    data transmission, 12
    ECG database, 13
    Fuzzy inference system, 16–18
    Fuzzy logics–based disease detection system, 15–16
    Fuzzy rule, 16–17
    Fuzzy system, 16
    MIT-BIH Arrhythmia database, 13
    noise removal from, 14–15
    trapezoidal membership function, 17
    triangular membership function, 17
  compression and transmission techniques, 7
  data accessed, 23
  ECG Android App, 6
  electrocardiogram (ECG)
    data collection and monitoring equipment, 4
    data transmission system, 3, 4
  electroencephalographic (EEG), 7
  Fuzzy knowledge representation, 18–19
    algorithm, 20–22
    fuzzy inference, 22–23
    weighted average (WA), 22
  health monitoring, 6
  healthcare, applications
    Centers for Disease Control and Prevention, 38
    health monitoring system, 34–37
    medicine observing, 45
    patients with heart disease, GPS positioning applications, 43–44
    pharmaceutical counterfeit device prediction, 46
    portable medicine, 42
    real-time observing, 46
    remote steady ECG checking, 37
    restorative waste management information, 46
    smart administration, 45
    smart service, 39
    smart wheelchair uses, 40–42
    telemedicine innovation, 37–38
    therapeutic tools, 45
    Web of things (WoT) advancement, 38
    well-being ID card, 44–45

MAC (media access control address), 33
   convention, 34
peregrination and smart healthcare
   carrier sense multiple access—collision avoidance (CSMA/CA), 33
   radio frequency (RF), 33
   TDMA (time-division multiple access), 33
   unmanned vehicles (UVs), 34
   WBAN (wireless body area network), 32–33
   Wireless Sensor Network (WSN), 34
results and discussion, 23–24
RFID (radio frequency identification)
   applications to assist elderly live independently, 39–40
   innovation, 39
   wristbands, utilizations of, 42–43
smart data acquisition and processing system
   automatic ECG monitoring system, 10
   ECG signal with standard fiducial points, 9
   electrode placement in body, 8
   measuring heartbeat, 11
   QRS complex, 9
   SpO2 measuring device, 11
   waves, 9
   ultrasonic images, 7
Body area network (BAN), 5

applications of RFID wristbands, 231–232
connected data sharing, 228
data analysis, 236
drug storage, 227
end-to-end network and moderateness, 235–236
exact costs and improvising patient experience, 235
fighting pharmaceutical error, 227–228
GPS positioning, 232–233
health ID card, 233–234
hygiene compliance, 235
medical emergency management, 226–227
medical instrumentation and drug pursue, 228
mobile medication, 231
PACU, anticipating the arrival of patients in, 234–235
patient information management, 226–227
real time location technology, 234
remote observing, 238
remote therapeutic assistance, 237
research, 237
RFID applications, 229
smart wheel-chair applications, 229–231
tracking and alarms, 236
working on research side, 238
world anti-kidnapping system, 228–229
Cyberphysical system (CPS), 160

C

Calcifying Epithelial Odontogenic Tumors (CEOT), 197–198
Cardiovascular disease (CVD), 3
Carrier sense multiple access—collision avoidance (CSMA/CA), 33
Challenges in healthcare
   accuracy and data overload, 177
   business model, 178
   cost, 177–178
   data privacy and security, 177
   mobility, 178
Cloud computing, 121
Computerized hospital
   alarm system, 229

D

Decision tree (DT)
   for big data analysis, 122–124
Devices in healthcare, 179
   charting, 180
   patient and staff behavior tracking appliances, 180

E

Electrocardiogram (ECG)
   data collection and monitoring equipment, 4
   data transmission system, 3, 4
Electroencephalographic (EEG), 7

Index

G
Genetic algorithm (GA), 108–109

H
Healthcare, applications
  Centers for Disease Control and Prevention, 38
  health monitoring system, 34–37
  medicine observing, 45
  patients with heart disease, GPS positioning applications, 43–44
  pharmaceutical counterfeit device prediction, 46
  portable medicine, 42
  real-time observing, 46
  remote steady ECG checking, 37
  restorative waste management information, 46
  smart administration, 45
  smart service, 39
  smart wheelchair uses, 40–42
  telemedicine innovation, 37–38
  therapeutic tools, 45
  Web of things (WoT) advancement, 38
  well-being ID card, 44–45

I
Internet of Things (IoT), 46, 159
  advanced smart medical, 49
  application software, 121–122
  battling pharmaceutical error, 48
  benefits in healthcare
    data assortment and analysis, 179
    good patient experience, 179
    home care service, 179
    real-time monitoring, 178
    tracking and alerts, 179
  brain–computer interface (BCI), 71
  challenges in healthcare
    accuracy and data overload, 177
    business model, 178
    cost, 177–178
    data privacy and security, 177
    mobility, 178
  cloud computing, 121
  critical survey, discussion, 72
  cyberphysical system (CPS), 160
  dataset used EEG recordings, 73–79
  decision tree (DT)
    for big data analysis, 122–124
  depression, 70
  depression and machine learning, 81–83
  devices in healthcare, 179
    charting, 180
    patient and staff behavior tracking appliances, 180
  emerging role, 130
    artificial intelligence (AI), 132
    background study, 133–134
    challenges, 131
    connectivity, 132
    data processing/data mining, 132
    devices, 131
    sensors, 132
    user interface, 133
  fMRI and EEG signals, 71
  health management
    blood pressure observation, 169
    body temperature monitoring, 169
    electrocardiogram (ECG) observation, 168
    glucose level sensing, 168
    oxygen saturation observation, 169
  for healthcare, 164–165
    utility and applications for, 166–169
  healthcare security, 169, 172
    ambient intelligence, 176
    augmented reality, 176
    big data, 175–176
    cloud computing, 175
    grid computing, 175
    networks, 176
    security challenges, 173–174
    security necessity, 173
    wearables, 176
  machine learning (ML)
    model, 84–88
    techniques, 71
  medical equipment and medication control, 167
  medical information system
    blood information management, 167
    emergency system, 166–167

information sharing, 167
  patient information management, 166
  storage management of medication, 166
medication storage management, 47–48
methods used
  connected medical/health devices, 144
  M-health, 143–144
  monitoring in-patients' health, 138–139
  nursing system, 136–138
  optimizing care, 139–142
  targeted field, communication scenario in, 135–136
  tele-health, 142–143
middleware, 120–121
M2M communication, 160
  architectural view, 162–164
  dominant parts of, 164
  general framework of, 161
mobile medical and telemedicine care
  mobile medical care, 168
  telemedicine, service, 168
persistent statistics management, 47
quiet information management, 48
radio frequency identification (RFID), 118–119
reports and approaches used, 134–135
restorative device and pharmaceuticals anticounterfeiting, 48–49
seizure formation and depression, 80–81
smart medicinal management, 47
smartphone-based healthcare app, 171–172
therapeutic waste information management, 49
utilizations for healthcare, 170
wireless sensor network (WSN), 120, 160

K

Knowledge discovery in databases (KDD), 101–102

M

MAC (media access control address), 33
  convention, 34
Machine learning (ML)
  model, 84–88
  techniques, 71
Medical information system
  blood information management, 167
  emergency system, 166–167
  information sharing, 167
  patient information management, 166
  storage management of medication, 166
M2M communication, 160
  architectural view, 162–164
  dominant parts of, 164
  general framework of, 161

O

Odontogenic tumors, IoT
  ameloblastic fibroma, 197
  Calcifying Epithelial Odontogenic Tumors (CEOT), 197–198, 203
  in India, prevalence of
    adenomatoid odontogenic tumor, 196–197
    ameloblastoma, 195
    odontoma, 196
  medical diagnosis, 187–189
  odontogenic myxoma, 198
  pathogenesis, 190
    WHO classification, 190–194
  squamous odontogenic tumor, 203–204
    adenomatoid odontogenic tumor, 201
    ameloblastic fibroma, 201–202
    ameloblastoma, 198–199
    anatomical site of distribution, 199
    odontogenic myxoma, 202–203
    odontoma, 200
    peripheral ameloblastoma, 200
  WHO classification (1971)
    benign odontogenic tumor, 190–191
    malignant odontogenic tumors, 191
  WHO classification (1992)
    benign odontogenic tumor, 191–192
    malignant odontogenic tumors, 192
  WHO classification (2005)
    benign odontogenic tumor, 192–193
    malignant odontogenic tumors, 193
  WHO classification (2017)
    benign odontogenic tumor, 193–194
    malignant odontogenic tumors, 194

Index

P
Post-Anesthesia Care Unit (PACU), 235

Q
QRS complex, 9

R
Relevant current applications of IoT
  benefits
    improved client engagement, 209
    improvisation of technologies, 209–210
    reduced waste, 210
  biomedical engineering, 220
    aims and scope, 221–222
  computerized hospital
    alarm system, 229
    applications of RFID wristbands, 231–232
    connected data sharing, 228
    data analysis, 236
    drug storage, 227
    end-to-end network and moderateness, 235–236
    exact costs and improvising patient experience, 235
    fighting pharmaceutical error, 227–228
    GPS positioning, 232–233
    health ID card, 233–234
    hygiene compliance, 235
    medical emergency management, 226–227
    medical instrumentation and drug pursue, 228
    mobile medication, 231
    PACU, anticipating the arrival of patients in, 234–235
    patient information management, 226–227
    real time location technology, 234
    remote observing, 238
    remote therapeutic assistance, 237
    research, 237
    RFID applications, 229
    smart wheel-chair applications, 229–231
    tracking and alarms, 236
    working on research side, 238
    world anti-kidnapping system, 228–229
  evaluation, 208–209
  future, scope
    artificial learning (AL), 212
    cybercriminals, 211–212
    DDOS assaults, 214
    5G networks, 213
    5G'S arrival, 214
    routers, 213
    security and privacy considerations, 214
    urban people, 212
    vehicles, 213–214
  practical applications
    energy management, 211
    enterprise, 210
    health fix health monitor, 210
    massive scale deployment, 211
    medical and healthcare, 210
    nest reasonable thermostat, 210
    personal home automation system, 210
    utilities, 211
    WeMo switch reasonable plug, 210
  R&D group, 215–218
    literature survey, 219–220
  special applications, 222–223
    anti-counterfeiting, therapeutic device and professionally, 225
    complete timeframe observing, 225
    and management, 223–224
    medical instrumentation and drug watching, 223–224
    restorative waste information management, 226
  specialized issues facing medical
    in biomedical, utilizations of, 241
    cost, 240–241
    data compression, 239
    data security, 239
    dynamic networking, 239
    healthcare charting, 242
    hearables zone, 241
    information over-burden and precision, 240
    ingestible sensors, 241
    knowledge completeness, 239

moodables locale, 242
and node quality management, 239
numerous devices, 240
PC vision innovation, 242
RFID (radio frequency identification)
  applications to assist elderly live
    independently, 39–40
  innovation, 39
  wristbands, utilizations of, 42–43

S

Smart healthcare, explicit applications in IoT
  alert area, 55
  associated information sharing, 51
  battling pharmaceutical error, 51
  medicinal apparatus and drug tracking, 51
  medicinal backup administration, 50
  patient data management, 49–50
  protein structure, prediction of, 52–55
  quiet evidence controlling, 50
Smart hospitals, IOT, 144
  analytics and the use of big data, 151–152
  big data analytics and, 152
    bioinformation, 153
    clinical information, 154
    neuroinformatics, 153–154
  clinical efficiency tasks, 146
  data, privacy and security of, 150–151
  natural calamities and disasters, 151
  operations efficiency, 145
  patient well-being, 146–147
  stages, 148–150
Specialized issues confronting, IoT
  brain-tumor detection, 59–64
  duplicate medicine detection, 58–59
  information completeness and data compression, 56–57
  node versatility and dynamic large scale system, 55–56
Squamous odontogenic tumor, 203–204
  adenomatoid odontogenic tumor, 201
  ameloblastic fibroma, 201–202
  ameloblastoma, 198–199

anatomical site of distribution, 199
odontogenic myxoma, 202–203
odontoma, 200
peripheral ameloblastoma, 200
State-of-the-art survey on decision trees IoT, 100
  advantages of DT, 105–106
  artificial neural network (ANN), 111–112
  big data analysis, 112–113
  collection of data, 114
  commerce and business, big data in, 116–117
  consuming and visualizing, 115
  data analysis, traditional approach for, 112
  data mining, 101–102, 103
  decision tree (DT), 103–104
  four V's, 113
  fuzzy application in modeling, 109–110
  genetic algorithm (GA), 108–109
  healthcare sector, big data, 117
  induction of decision tree (DT), 104–105
  issues in big data, 115
  knowledge discovery in databases (KDD), 101–102
  limitations, 112
  processing and analyzing, 115
  scientific research, big data in, 116
  social network, big data analytics in, 115–116
  society administration, big data, 117–118
  soft computing aspects in DT, 107–108
  storing, 114
  tree pruning, 106–107

T

TDMA (time-division multiple access), 33

U

Ultrasonic images, 7
Unmanned vehicles (UVs), 34

W

WBAN (wireless body area network), 32–33
Web of things (WoT) advancement, 38
Weighted average (WA), 22
Well-being ID card, 44–45
WHO classification (1971)
  benign odontogenic tumor, 190–191
  malignant odontogenic tumors, 191
WHO classification (1992)
  benign odontogenic tumor, 191–192
  malignant odontogenic tumors, 192
WHO classification (2005)
  benign odontogenic tumor, 192–193
  malignant odontogenic tumors, 193
WHO classification (2017)
  benign odontogenic tumor, 193–194
  malignant odontogenic tumors, 194
Wireless Sensor Network (WSN), 34